I0619962

OUR JOURNEY

A True Story About Caregiving:
The Good, the Bad, and the *Really* Ugly

Cassie Abel

Acknowledgements

I want to thank my family and friends for their support during my caregiving journey with my mother. Without their encouragement and love, none of this would have been possible.

I want to thank our "Weekday Warriors", our caregivers for whom having Mom at home would not have been possible without. Angie, Cassi, Alishea, Sydney, Joanna, Kizzy, Maggie, and Pam your love and dedication to my mother was truly a blessing.

I want to thank our hospice nurses, Charlotte, Judy, and Ashton, who gave me understanding and comfort in our most crucial times.

I want to thank my nephew, Wesley, for creating the cover art for this book. Your grandmother was so very proud of your artistry, and I am honored to have it shown on my first publication.

I want to thank my editor, Christi, for her guidance, encouragement, and friendship. From the moment you sang as Simba during class in middle school, to becoming my sounding board in this crazy idea to write a book, thank you for everything.

For Scott, Emma, and Archer.
I would never have made it without you.
I love you all so much.
Thank you for being right by my side on this journey.

This is for every caregiver who finds a piece of themselves within these chapters.

In loving memory of my first best friend, my mother.
I love you.
I love you more.
Impossible.

Introduction

In May of 2020, when the world was crumbling with COVID, my world was crumbling with another lettered disease that would forever alter the path of my life: ALS.

Amyotrophic Lateral Sclerosis (ALS) is a rare, progressive, and fatal neurological disease that primarily affects the nerve cells responsible for controlling voluntary muscle movement, such as chewing, walking, and talking. It affects all the nerve cells in the brain and spinal cord. People with ALS lose their ability to walk, talk, eat, and eventually breathe. There is no cure or treatment that halts ALS. In a nutshell, ALS is among the three "baddies" of neurological diseases, right up there with Parkinsons and Alzheimer's. In a nutshell *within* a nutshell, it's *fucking* ruthless, unfair, and unobjective of who it targets. ALS typically strikes people between the ages of 40 and 70.

My mother was just shy of her 71st birthday when she was *officially* diagnosed; however, it was just after her 70th birthday that she began the diagnostic process because we knew something wasn't right with her body. Numerous falls, loss of strength in her legs, and other red flags had risen slowly between the end of 2018 and the summer of 2019, her symptoms gaining in intensity until she was finally diagnosed with ALS in the spring of 2020.

After years of battling, preparing, and accepting her fate, my mother declined to the point that she was no longer safe alone in her home and had begun to look at skilled nursing facilities. Instead, my family opted to welcome her into our new home, and things changed rapidly for all of us. For fifteen months, I (along with a team of weekday aides) performed as my mother's caregiver. She had 24/7 care from the moment she moved into our home. It was this home that we had worked hard to make accessible for her.

For fifteen months I watched as her body continue to fail her over and over. I felt every emotion known to man, perhaps even some that have yet to be named. From anger and depression to joy and peace, I'd been strapped into an emotional roller coaster that took a toll on my body as well as my soul. It was then I decided to share our journey.

I began a personal blog about two months before she moved in. I knew there were going to be many ups and downs. I knew it was important for me to have an outlet to allow myself to feel and process everything. I kept the blog private for about a year before deciding to make it available to others.

I belong to quite a number of online ALS communities, and we would share tips and tricks for taking care of our PALS (Person with ALS). We would also share with each other our fears and frustrations as CALS (Caregiver for someone with ALS). The guilt we felt for the anger, abandonment, stress, every emotion that made us feel like worthless human beings was something we all had in common. Here we were, healthier than our PALS who, for the most part, couldn't do anything for themselves. Because if they could, believe me—they would. Who were we to have these feelings? We signed up for caregiving, but our people did not sign up for their disease. Who did we think we were?

I have that answer.
Humans.
We are *human*.

We are allowed to feel every beautiful or hideous thing that comes along with whatever decisions we make, whether for ourselves or for others. It doesn't always mean rainbows and sunshine, happy-go-lucky, 'look at the wonderful thing we are doing for the person we love.'

No. That also includes the anger, the resentment, the regret, the depression, the worry, the anxiety. That includes the good, the bad, and the *really* ugly.

That is why I had decided to take my writing public, turning my online journal into this book. I want to not only educate other caregivers about tips and tricks that work in many common situations, but also share that what we feel is *exactly* how we are supposed to feel. We are not alone. *You* are not alone.

What defines you as a caregiver? In short, a caregiver is a person who tends to the needs or concerns of a person with both short and long-term limitations due to illness, injury, or disability.

I share my family's journey for those out there who are, have been, or will be a caregiver.

As much as this is a journey for those ill with the disease, disability, or injury, this is *our* journey too, and you should know you deserve to have your needs and concerns tended to as well.

You cannot pour from an empty well.
You cannot give what you do not have.

Energy, trust, compassion, and support—these are all things you give that you also must be able to receive in return, whether from a community or from within yourself.

With much love, support, encouragement, and understanding to all you Caregiving Warriors out there, you have this... even when you don't.

Cassie N. Abel

CHAPTER 1:
"I'm going to call you 'Weeble-Wobble,' the way you're walking!"

There is a photo of me and Momma, a simple selfie from a work conference back in 2019. Just another selfie we'd taken, yet that photo had quite the meaning behind it. And at the same time, it really didn't. We happened to be at a conference together, having dinner before a full schedule of meetings the next day. Nothing unusual about any of that. Yet within six months' time, this photo would signify the beginning of a journey that neither one of us could even fathom would become our lives.

In May of 2019, my mom and I attended a conference for the company we both worked for. At this time my mom lived an hour from where I lived, so we didn't see one another except maybe every other weekend or so. At this conference, the meeting hall was quite a walk from the lobby of the hotel. I distinctly remember walking with my mother from the lobby toward the meeting hall and raising an eyebrow at the way she was walking.

She would move side to side as she walked, as if her hips were uneven. I remember asking her what was wrong, what hurt, and she replied, "I'm not sure, I must have pulled something in my back maybe."

If only it had been that simple. I didn't think much of it then—I mean, she was almost 70 and had suffered from back issues in the past. She didn't seem to be in pain, didn't seem concerned. So, why should I worry?

"I'm going to call you 'Weeble-Wobble,' the way you're walking!" I joked with her. I remember this *vividly*. I remember the look of the long corridor we were walking through, the outfit she was wearing, the sound of her voice as she laughed at my joke.

"Weeble-Wobble" would be something I called her for the next few months.

She would weeble-wobble as we walked the mall.
She would weeble-wobble when we took my kids to the park.

I called her Weeble-Wobble at her surprise 70th Birthday that summer.

We would tease about her 'getting up there' in age and her weebling and her wobbling.

Even when she had her first fall only a month after that conference. She didn't get hurt, just 'tripped' at the airport. She brushed it off. "That was weird, I must be wearing the wrong shoes. You know me being a Weeble-Wobble and all."

We joked.
We laughed.

Then, a few short months later, we stopped.

We stopped joking.
We stopped laughing.

By November of 2019, life for my mother took a very sharp and twisted turn.

CHAPTER 2:
Momma

To create a complete image of the relationship between me and my "Momma" isn't simple because she is *not* a simple woman. She had two boys prior to me and married my father, who had five children of his own (three boys, two girls). By the time I was created between them, my siblings were teenagers. This meant that even though I have seven siblings, I primarily grew up as an only child. My relationship with my Momma is idyllic–the kind you read about in stories of wonderful childhoods. Which makes sense considering I had a wonderful childhood. Momma had worked as a nurse and nursing home administrator, took care of me when I was sick, made sure I had home-cooked meals, and always kept the house clean. She taught me the importance of tidiness, good grades, morals, values… the whole nine yards. All were lessons that would continue even through my college and young adult years.

I cannot remember a time my mother and I had a huge disagreement. Nothing more than the typical, "she's old, she doesn't understand." My Momma pushed me toward a higher education, pushed me when I wanted to quit. She is always my number one supporter. My Momma got me through my divorce. My Momma got me through my miscarriage. My Momma was the first to cheer me on at every graduation and was right by my side when I found out I had passed my boards and became a Health Facility Administrator. My Momma is the first person I call when I have any news of joy or sadness. My Momma and I have spoken or texted on the phone every single day since cell phones became a thing.

In short, my Momma is my *very best* friend.

She grew up as the eldest of five girls. Back in the 1950s and 1960s, her family didn't have much of anything. She has recalled many stories of wearing rags and getting bullied at school for her Coke-bottle glasses, worn shoes, and tattered clothing. Being the oldest, she also was set to being a "second mother" to her sisters. She learned to cook and clean at a very young age, ensuring the whole family was taken care of when her mother was working or unable to do so. Momma was married young, as were most back in those times, and although the marriage was neither easy nor charming, she did come away with two sons from that marriage.

Momma worked through high school and then beauty school. Around the time she met my father, she aspired to become a nurse, so she did. She became an LPN at age 33, and the photo of her at her graduation, pregnant with me, has always been one of my favorites. She returned to schooling when she was almost 50 years old to obtain her Health Facility Administrator license and became an administrator of skilled nursing facilities. She still works in close capacity with them to this day, despite the difficult turn her life has taken.

It was a career path that I followed as well, although I never became a nurse. I worked for 18 years as a marketing director for skilled nursing facilities, receiving my bachelor's in public relations and then my administrator's license when I was 36 years old.

Not only is my Momma my best friend, she is my mentor in both life and career.

CHAPTER 3:
Surprise! Happy 70th Birthday!

June of 2019

I planned and executed a surprise birthday party for my mom. She had never really celebrated a birthday, and this was a *big* one. I had to fabricate an excuse for her to travel the hour south to my house from hers, mainly stating I wanted to take her out to eat with my two brothers. That wasn't the hard part. The hard part was wanting to blindfold her and trying to give her a reason as to why. The only thing I could come up with was a lie that one of my brothers had something really cool they wanted to show her outside his home but wanted to keep it a surprise. I guess it wasn't *too* much of a lie!

In the early spring, just a few months before this birthday party, my mother had semi-retired as a nursing home administrator. This was when I became an administrator of the nursing home she had served. She continued to work as a nursing home consultant, but after 20 years, she decided to give herself a break and semi-retire. She was ready to relax, travel, and celebrate her "golden years."

Her 70th birthday party was such a success! Surprised as she was, we even have a few photos of her crying in happiness and joy. She had friends she'd worked with for over 20 years there. She had all four of her sisters and their families there, most of whom she hadn't seen in quite some time. Six of her children were there with all of their kids and their kids and grandkids.

It. Was. Fabulous.

At this time, Mom was still Weeble-Wobble. I remember we had to help her into my van, and then we had to hold onto her as we led her inside the event room. Still, she was able to move around and walk the entire day with only a little weebling and wobbling. Still no huge cause for concern.

This day is truly a memory I know I'll always cherish, and I'm so glad she was able to celebrate this birthday with so many of her friends and family. No one knew what the future had in store for us, and not just with her health. We were a mere six months away from a global health crisis and all that came with it.

CHAPTER 4:
Mother-Daughter Vacation

Labor Day Weekend 2019

During Labor Day weekend of 2019, Momma and I went on a mother-daughter get-away to Nashville, Tennessee. She had mentioned earlier in the year how she'd always wanted to stay at the Opryland Hotel. She had wanted a room that overlooked the waterfalls inside. So, I made it happen! Never thought of how *not* great of an idea it would be to visit Nashville on Labor Day weekend, but we did it anyway—and had a *blast* alongside the bachelorette parties and all! Mom and I took so many photos of us on our balcony looking over the waterfalls that we dubbed it a photo-shoot. Many of the pictures of her from that weekend became my absolute favorites of her.

When my mother was finally diagnosed, I remember going back in my mind and recalling the warning signs. At the time, we didn't know they were warning signs, but it was obvious in retrospect. This trip had a few of those instances. At this point in 2019, my mom was still Weeble Wobble, except it had gotten worse. She would rock side to side as she walked, and she was starting to experience some pain in her hips and lower back. My mother, the nurse, of course had yet to call her physician, but there was now a twinge of concern. It wasn't clear, though, because she was able to walk the entire length of the Opryland Mall. Was she slower? Sure. However, she had just turned 70.

What did stand out about this trip was the moment I realized she wasn't able to walk up the stairs anymore. Mom could take a few steps, but when it came to either taking stairs or the elevator, she needed the elevator every time, which was unlike her. At one part of the hotel, the elevator was out of service, so we had no choice but to use the stairs. There were ten steps, then a platform, then another ten steps.

The concern started for me here. Holding on to her arm as she walked up the stairs in a way I had never seen her do before. She'd have to side swipe her leg up one and hold on to me and the rail to get the other up. I remember the sounds of the waterfalls in the distance suddenly was lost in the roar of my heart beating in my chest. Mom brushed it off some, saying she should probably get her hips looked at. She thought she'd slipped a disc or pulled something. Even then, the small amount of concern wasn't enough for me to push her.

I wish I had pushed her.

Another part of this trip that stands out in hindsight is when we were waiting to ride the trolley that would take us on a tour of downtown Nashville. There was a younger lady waiting with an elderly woman in a wheelchair. The younger lady told us she was a friend of the elderly lady and the lady always wanted to go to Nashville. Mom and I watched her take care of the lady in the wheelchair. I vividly remember my mom leaning over and saying, "Think you'll take care of me one day? When I'm not able to do it myself, you'll still take me places and make sure I'm okay?"

I smiled at her and said, "Well, duh, of course I will, Momma."

Never did I imagine just how true that promise would become in the *very* near future.

CHAPTER 5:
Summertime Sleepover

Summer 2019

One afternoon in the late summer of 2019, I took my children the hour north to visit Momma. It was a "sleep-over" weekend, so we went to the park to play, went out to eat, and slept over at her house. I captured Mom on the swings with my four-year-old son, swinging seriously high off the ground. In one photo, they're both in mid-air, looking at each other with brilliant smiles on their faces.

It's hard to articulate what it means to have this photo of my son looking at his grandmother with so much love as they laughed and swung. At the time, I loved it merely because it was cute. But as I look at it now, there's a twinge of pain in my heart and a whole lot of frustration associated with it.

ALS isn't fair.

I mean, what disease really is? During this process I've watched this disease take so much from my mother very quickly. It's physically painful for her and very emotionally painful for me to watch. There's another aspect though that rips my heart to shreds... my children.

ALS is taking my children's grandmother, and they are too young to understand the significance of it. Children are resilient. They have such innocent and sugar-coated expectations of life. My mother has gone from being able to take them for sleepovers and swing with them at the park to being permanently in a wheelchair, and my children have accepted the changes better than anyone could have imagined.

It's me who's been struggling with acceptance—watching from afar, seeing everything they'll be missing, feeling the heartache as my daughter talks to my mother about her wedding when she grows up. The gut-wrenching reality is that my mom and I both know she won't physically be here to see it.

Thoughts like this are what I try to shake away from the 'thought bank.' Not because I'm in denial—the opposite, in fact. I know what's coming. My mother does too.

I just wish she could have swung happily on those swings for so many more years. I wish that when those photos were taken, we could have had even a glimpse of what the next few months had in store. We had no idea. No clue.

Chapter 6:
Let's Talk Falls

June of 2019

Mom had her very first fall.

She was at the airport after having vacationed in Las Vegas with her life-partner, a man who came into her life after my father had passed. He became the one who would be by her side during her retirement years and ride this journey with her as well.

One minute she was walking inside the airport, the next she was staring up from the ground. I remember her calling me after it had happened.

"You fell!?" I repeated into the phone. "What the heck?"

My mom went on to say she had bought some new shoes during vacation, and she was fairly certain those are what made her fall. She didn't injure herself, fortunately—just a few bumps and bruises. I remember both of us thinking it was just a weird thing to happen.

Weebles are supposed to Wobble, but they aren't supposed to fall down.

In July of 2019, my mom had her *second* fall.

She was once again on vacation. This time was with her sister, and they were in Memphis at a casino. This fall was harder than the first and just as sudden. Although she didn't have a serious injury, she was very sore and bruised after this fall. When she called me, my heart *sank* in my chest. "You fell *again*!?"

This time there wasn't any laughter, even when she replied, "I think it's these damn shoes!"

I asked if it was the same pair she'd been wearing in Vegas, but it wasn't. They were different. Now comes my concern. She agreed she needed to get in to the doctor at some point, but she hadn't made the appointment. 'There's more fun to be had,' she said. Once the vacations she had planned were done, then she'd go.

Thinking back after we had received her diagnosis, we realized what these two falls were.

Symptoms.
Signs.
Foot drop.

After the second incident, she started to have falls at home. I got frequent text messages with photos of scraped knees, bruised elbows, etc. She'd lost her footing, or she'd tripped. The frequency increased, and each time it would be harder for her to get up from the fall.

By winter of 2019, she started to use a rolling walker at her home to get around, because her foot drop became so pronounced that she could hardly lift her feet off the ground when she took a step.

Her condition continued to deteriorate throughout the rest of that year. The disease we didn't yet know she had was causing her muscles to atrophy and leaving her severely debilitated. We learned later on that falls can actually worsen, or speed up, the ALS disease process, making it more difficult to heal each time—which is exactly what happened to her.

CHAPTER 7:
What We THOUGHT We Knew

The End of 2019

On December 1st of 2019, my family decided to do a Thankmas. We have a large extended family, so instead of people trying to figure out who can do Thanksgiving or Christmas, plus making sure my mom didn't have to do all the hosting, we came up with Thankmas. We rented a banquet hall (the one we had used for Mom's birthday party), and everyone pitched in, bringing the food, handling the games, and doing the present portion.

Due to the increasing number of falls my mom had experienced the previous few months, her balance wasn't as good and that was now *very* apparent. She was still able to drive, but she had to physically lift her legs into the car. And yes, it was scary that she was actually still driving. We still didn't know what was going on, but at this point we knew *something* was wrong.

I no longer joked about it or called her Weeble Wobble.

Mom had gone to her physician, and they had ordered blood work, MRIs, and CT scans of her back and neck, trying to determine why she was losing her strength in her legs. She was 70 years old, but this was *far* from anything to do with advancing age. None of the results provided an answer.

It would be after this Thankmas that her physician would meet with her about performing an EMG. This test, performed by a neurologist, would start to point us in a direction we never knew we'd go. While administering the test, the doctor told her, "We cannot confirm this, but to me, it looks like ALS."

I'll never forget that phone call from her. She was crying so hard. I kept telling her that maybe they were wrong, but the test confirmed her muscles in both legs were dying and likely causing her falls. It even revealed that she was losing some muscle in her arms and neck.

21

"It's what it is, Cassie. I just know it," she cried.

I was outside in our backyard, phone pressed tightly against my ear as I listened to the strongest woman in the world cry. But I couldn't get myself to even shed a tear. After calling my sister, who practically wailed at the news, I kept wondering why I didn't feel this sudden surge of grief. I believe I was in shock, denial, and disbelief that such an ugly disease could be attacking the person in the world I love the most. That just didn't happen.

Diagnosing ALS is not a short or fast process. Although the EMG showed significant evidence that this was what we were dealing with, she would have to have another EMG performed in a few months' time to really get a confirmation.

Maybe it wasn't ALS. Maybe it was something that actually has a cure. Maybe she just needed a little surgery. Maybe she needed another regime of drugs.

Maybe.
Maybe.
Maybe.

I was counting on so many maybes because I am always a 'silver lining' type of person. I am an optimist. I'm obsessed with positivity in my life. But I still felt that twinge in the pit of my stomach. I knew. I didn't show it. I didn't express it. But I knew.

What we didn't know, in December of 2019, was just how crazier our lives were about to get.

CHAPTER 8:
Hindsight

Beginning of 2020

It's easier to *analyze* and *evaluate* situations when we're recalling them, rather than when we're experiencing them.

If that isn't an accurate summation of what 2020 would bring, I don't know what is. 2020 started off halfway decent. Normal. Did we hear about things happening over in China? Sure. Were the majority of Americans worried? Not *yet*. It was being stated in the media that it was coming for us, as early as December of 2019. Americans are good at denial too. There's a parallel to be drawn there. For my family, 2020 was a promise to a better year, as is the hope with every turn of the New Year.

In January, my mother was becoming progressively weaker. She stopped driving (thank *God*), as it was very difficult for her to lift her foot from gas to brake. She was still having to physically pull her legs into the vehicle, and we had to lift from under her knees to push her the rest of the way back into the passenger seat.

Her physician had started her on some medications to help with sleep and pain; none of which were really working. By this time, considering our professional backgrounds, my mother and I knew she had ALS. We had to wait for her second EMG in a few months to confirm, but everything else had been ruled out and she was having every symptom. Weakness, foot drop, twinges, aches, just *everything*.

In February, my mother had a devastating loss; her Yorkie, Bailey, had died due to old age. Oh, that broke her heart, and my heart broke for her. She took it especially hard because not only was her own body failing her and this new reality was crashing down, but now she didn't have her little fur baby anymore. She spent most of her days by herself in the house, and Bailey had been a companion for her. Now he is gone.

Mom had also been having even more falls, always unable to get up on her own. She was using a rolling walker to get from point A to point B. I watched as she transported herself to the bathroom, her arms shaking while trying to hold her balance. Each time she'd tell me, "This is going pretty fast, isn't it?"

It was.

I recall her telling me about a repairman that was coming to the house. Mom was sitting in her chair and needed to get something from the table. The table was by a bay of windows at the front of the house. Mom lost her footing and fell to the floor. No one else was home. She couldn't move to sit herself up, nor did she have the strength to 'army crawl' to her cell phone. It was a few moments later when the doorbell rang, signaling that the repairman was there for his service call. Mom started to call out and eventually the young man looked through the bay windows, seeing my mother on the floor.

The repairman started to panic, asking if she was hurt and if he needed to call 911. Mom was able to talk to him, saying she wasn't hurt but she couldn't move. The young man asked if the door was unlocked, and of course it wasn't. But Mom remembered that the windows were unlocked, and one was slightly open. The man worked himself through the small opening and was able to lift the rest of the window up, crawling through and helping her back to her chair.

This was a desperate moment for my mother. Far beyond embarrassment, there was now fear creeping into her mind (and mine, when she told me about it). It was at that moment I went and bought Mom an Apple Watch and set myself as her emergency contact (along with her life-partner and my brother). If she fell, we'd be alerted. If she was unable to talk to us through the watch, we could contact emergency personnel to reach her much faster than we could. Technology really is a life saver at times.

On March 7th, we went to visit my mother for the weekend. Up to this point, I'd been going almost every other weekend. We got out of the house, went to eat, and then went to the pet shop. Mom just wanted to love on some puppies, since she was missing her Bailey. I remember having to help her out of the van, walking alongside her with my arms supporting her, as she could not walk without assistance. It was difficult because I was afraid I was going to drop her.

Little did I know that this would be the last time I saw my mother for months. *Months!*

At this time, I was working as a Nursing Home Administrator. The following week would be the very beginning of pure hell and exhaustion as COVID made its way into the US. The Centers for Medicare and Medicaid Services (CMS) would officially bring the hammer down, and on March 10th, we would have to lock the doors of the nursing home. In fact, the whole world was shutting down.

With the pandemic starting to be taken seriously and schools and businesses being shut down, I decided that in no way, shape, or form would I be allowing myself to possibly bring something like COVID to my ailing mother.

So, I stayed away.

I became so slammed at work as well as having to reconfigure things at home (since my daughter's school was closed) that I was lucky to talk to my mother every other day for quite a long time.

It was terrible. The timing, like everything else that circled around COVID, couldn't have been worse.

Chapter 9:
The Official Diagnosis

May 2020

It was official.

The results of mom's second EEG confirmed what we had suspected for months:

ALS

Although we'd known it in our hearts, hearing the official results was another blow. It confirmed that this was going to be her reality, that her future would be shorter than it should ever have to be. It was going to be painful. It was going to be devastating.

I listened to my mother grieve for what she would lose, and we cried together. This time, there was no shock value. My pain came throttling from my throat as I sobbed. Hearing her say the words, "I just wish I could get it over with and go out with a massive coronary or stroke." No daughter wants to hear that; however, I understood exactly where my mom was coming from.

Strong.
Independent.
Fierce.
Brave.
Stubborn.
Inspiring.

All of those words exemplify who my mother had always been and would continue to be. To have a diagnosis such as ALS that, no matter what you do or who you are, takes and takes and takes until there's nothing left. It's beyond unfair. Don't get me wrong, it's not fair for *anyone,* no matter who they are. But this is *my* mother, and I'm allowed to stomp my feet and cry into the night about how unfair this is. For her. For me. I'm allowed to feel selfish—even if just for a bit, even if only in private.

My mother's period of selfishness was brief as well. She stomped her feet (well, figuratively) and cried – and then sucked it up and dealt with it. That was something she had always instilled in me growing up and even in my adult years:

"Suck it up and deal. Sure, it's hard and you have a right to feel the pain, frustration, and agony... but you don't get to live there. You don't allow it to swallow you. Instead, you suck it up and move on. You find ways around that barrier. Was it not how you planned? Too bad, because that's how it is now. How are you going to make it work for you?"

When I tell you how amazing my mother is, I mean it. Anyone who has ever met my mother will tell you the same. I'm not blowing rainbows and sunshine—I'm telling you my mother is the *most* amazing human being you will *ever* meet, and I have the honor of being her daughter.

Chapter 10:
Happy Birthday, Mom

June 2020

The silver lining of getting her official ALS diagnosis was that she could now start seeing ALS specialists and going to the ALS clinics. She would be able to get the equipment she needed, including the snazzy, 400-pound motorized wheelchair. It wasn't much of a silver lining, but it was something.

Although she was just now getting her diagnosis, due to the way her body had continued to fail her, my mother was prepared. She'd always been prepared in all aspects of her life. Before the official diagnosis, she was already ordering a Hoyer lift, even though she was still transporting herself (painfully) to and from the places she wanted to go. She ordered herself a hospital bed and kept it stored for the time she knew she'd eventually need it. Coming from a healthcare background, especially nursing, my mother knew what her future held for her.

In this situation, no matter the sudden onset of injury, disability, or illness, many are unable to gather the means or resources needed to get prepared and have the equipment they need to function. It is a sad reality in our country. There are not enough resources. There is never enough money. This was something my mother and I would face in the near future.

For Mom's 71st birthday, in June of 2020, I said SCREW YOU COVID, and I went to see her. I hadn't seen her since March. Three months had gone by, and she'd been officially diagnosed since the last time I'd seen her. I hadn't gotten to see her in her snazzy new wheels. Yes, we talked on the phone quite a bit, but work was extremely hectic with the pandemic—though at this time, my nursing facility had yet to be hit. I did take precautions. I took a rapid test to ensure I was negative and wore a mask.

But let's be honest.

Although I did the rapid on myself and my children, we didn't stay 6ft apart. I hugged my mother. My kids hugged my mother. Because in the three months I had not seen her, *so much had changed.* Hearing about it over the phone was one thing, but seeing it in person was something else entirely. Who knew if or when we'd get the chance again? That could be said for anyone, but when you have a terminal illness, it becomes terrifyingly real.

Her ALS chair had finally arrived, and boy, that thing did everything but turn her upside down. She was so fast in it, was able to go up and down, and side to side. It was perfect. It was accessible.

It was so hard to see her in it.

In June of 2020, she was still able to wiggle off the chair and stand up on her feet to transfer to the toilet and her bed. It wasn't a pretty sight to see. Her arms trembled as she held onto the walker. Her feet, both experiencing drop foot, would drag as she pulled her legs. By the time she was done using the restroom and back in her wheelchair, her entire little body was shaking, and she was drenched in sweat.

But she did it. That was how she continued to remain as independent as she could. Seeing her like that was equal parts heartbreaking and inspiring.

In early August, I came to visit Mom again. When talking with her on the phone, she'd begun to mention how lonely she was. It was a subject that came up often. She would spend most of the day on her own while her partner ran errands and such. It was hard to get mom in and out of the house—I get that. But she was *so* bored and *so* lonely. She was so used to going and doing what she wanted, when she wanted. Now she couldn't.

I'd had enough.

I drove up that weekend to see my mother and I took her out. We went shopping at her favorite stores and then went out to eat. As frustrating as it can sometimes be to maneuver a motorized wheelchair through a crowd, it was fabulous to get her out in the sunshine and fresh air. The smile this trip put on her face was worth it.

CHAPTER 11:
Meeting Sammy

August 2020

Mom's dog, Bailey, had died at the beginning of 2020. She'd lost her 13-year-old companion, along with so much more thanks to her ALS progression. She was finally ready to open herself up to loving another dog. Although she wouldn't be able to get down on the floor, she made other necessary arrangements so that she could still reach him to put him in a bed and give him food and water. She was still able to get herself in and out of bed and into her chair, so she made certain she would be the one to get up with him in the middle of the night.

Mom was always so worried about putting more on anyone else, especially her life partner. If there was something she wanted to do, she'd do it for as long as she could, and half the time she wouldn't let him help.

So, I found Sammy for Mom, and we brought him to her at the end of August. He's a spunky, fluffy, cute-as-a-button, full-blooded Shih tzu. Sammy was a companion for her, something to look forward to each and every day. Momma's life had always been full of zest and perpetual motion, so having Sammy meant everything to her. He gave her a routine to sustain and–let's be honest–a sense of purpose she'd been gradually losing.

She had secured a playpen atop a table for him so he'd have a place to rest that she could still reach from her wheelchair. She was able to utilize the elevation features of the chair to get his water bowl and food, bringing them both to the kitchen table so he could eat and drink while she held him. Her partner was the one to take him outside when needed, but she did everything else.

The joy Sammy gives my mother is still so important. She loves that little dog so deeply, and I have to think she also recognizes the purpose he serves for her as well. When big, bad things are happening, it's the small, good things that make all the difference.

CHAPTER 12:
Breathing Trials

September 2020

In September of 2020, mom had a visiting respiratory therapist from the ALS clinic come to her home. They brought along a diagnostic machine to evaluate her breathing and oxygen levels.

It wasn't the best news.

Mom's output was severely low, meaning she was retaining too much CO_2 (which can be deadly). This meant that the ALS was moving into her diaphragm. When we inhale 100% oxygen, our bodies then diffuse the CO_2, and that's what we exhale. In Mom's case, she could inhale perfectly well, but the diaphragm was being weakened by the ALS. She could no longer expel the CO_2 properly, and it would eventually cause a plethora of problems.

This is also the very reason why someone with ALS should never be given oxygen via nasal cannula/mask, etc. This is something many do not realize, including EMS professionals.

If you're a person with ALS who is having trouble breathing (which is very common toward the later stages), many medical professionals will see your low oxygen saturation and want to slap an oxygen mask on you. It is important that you, your healthcare professionals (many are not accustomed to ALS), and your loved ones/caregivers are aware of the dangers of this.

The respiratory therapist brought a Trilogy Non-Invasive Ventilator for her to wear at night. The hope was it would help her rest, as she was having a terrible time sleeping, and would alleviate her fatigue during the day.

Unfortunately, it was so uncomfortable that she couldn't sleep at all. She wasn't feeling short of breath, so she decided not to wear it.

When she first started to use it, the humidifier wasn't attached properly, and it leaked causing her to feel as if she were drowning. Eventually, her arms would become too weak to be able to remove the mask and the anxiety of having something on her face that she couldn't remove for herself was far more terrifying than *actually* utilizing the machine for its intended purpose. The Trilogy would come in and out of play for the next few months, but to this day she still doesn't wear it.

CHAPTER 13:
This Year is Officially a Blur

Late 2020 to Early 2021

2020 was the longest and shortest year ever due to the pandemic and mom's progression. Since I was unable to see her as often as I normally would, her changes came as a gigantic shock to me every time I saw her.

By autumn so much had changed. For a while mom's progression had slowed. They'd told us that could happen and called it a plateau. Unfortunately, the plateau was a brief one. By the end of that year, Mom would be completely unable to transfer herself without the use of mobility aids, as her legs would be completely paralyzed. Her feet would be purple and swollen from loss of circulation, and they'd cause her pain no matter how often she had them up. She would use the assistance of a sit-to-stand lift to transfer between bed, chair, and toilet.

There was a brief time that Mom had used hand-pedals on her wheelchair van so that she could actually drive. The Sienna was very cool, very handy, and worth every penny to be able to take her out and about. But she wanted to drive and approached the task with her usual determination. She went and got lessons and was licensed to be able to drive using hand-paddles. She was *so* excited!

Then the winter hit.

COVID outbreaks were happening everywhere, including my nursing facility. From the very first of December until the New Year of 2021, my nursing home was ravaged by COVID. It is an experience I will never ever forget. I didn't see mom even a single time during December. I barely saw my husband and kids. 2020 took a lot out of everyone, but it was especially hard for nursing homes. Because COVID was so thick in our state, everything shut down yet again. At the time, my mom could drive herself anywhere, but she had nowhere to go.

In January 2021, things continued to progress with my mom.

She was starting to lose control of her trunk area, so she'd slump or have to catch herself from falling. She had to rely 100% on her partner to take her to the bathroom, give her a shower, and put her to bed. She wasn't able to turn herself over in bed, having to wake him up in the middle of the night to do so. She couldn't take care of Sammy in the middle of the night either. She wasn't resting, she began to lose her appetite, and she was in pain more often than not.

But she was still working from home as a consultant. It gave her something to do rather than sit around and look at Facebook all day.

For myself the new year had me making promises to myself. 2020 had taken so much out of me and my family that I vowed to get my priorities straight. As much as I loved my last 17 years in long term care, being a nursing home administrator was not something I wanted to continue to do while having two small children at home. Like so many other healthcare workers, I'd been giving so much of myself to my work that I had nothing left to give my family.

A career opportunity presented itself at our hospital, and I jumped on it. I was nervous, having done nothing but work in nursing homes. I took a chance, and they took a chance on *me*. I was offered the position. Same salary, better benefits, manageable hours, and so much less responsibility that I could actually be a wife, a mom, a friend, and a *human* again. Totally worth it. Actual work-life balance. Who would have thought?

February brought on even more changes with my mother.

Now her arms were starting to twitch, which is a sign the muscle is dying. She was losing strength in her arms and losing her grip in both hands. She was also miserable.

Miserable.

She was so lonely and wanted to be able to do so much more than she could. To be honest, I was ready too. I was tired of not being able to get away enough to take her places and to do things with her.

Her partner was wonderful, but he didn't ask for this any more than she did. Mom was frustrated with herself, and she vented those frustrations upon the only person she ever saw—him. That wasn't fair to either of them, but it especially wasn't fair for him.

It wasn't safe for him either as he wasn't as young as he once was. Mom had become completely dependent on transfers and daily care. While transferring her, he hurt his back. The possibility of him hurting himself further, or mom getting physically hurt in the process, it just wasn't going to work for the two of them living together anymore.

It was heartbreaking for all of us.

CHAPTER 14:
Coming Home; Full Circle

April 2021

In March of that year, Mom voiced her desire to come home, and I admitted I wanted that too. At the time, my husband and I still lived in our starter home. Three bedrooms, one bath… the kind of home where your washer/dryer is in your kitchen and your dining room is also your living room. We'd been wanting to move ever since our first child had been born, and we'd added a second by this point. But it was our home, and we'd done well with it. While there had been a few homes that came for sale that we'd looked at, none of them had really caught our eye.

One glorious day we found a home for sale that we loved. It had four bedrooms, two and a half bathrooms, and plenty of space. It was perfect for our children to grow up in. Plenty of room for them to run and play and to have their own space. It was in a safe neighborhood within the same school district they already went to. It also had a fantastic kitchen, which I was *really* excited about.

Interesting tidbit: this house is my childhood home!

My parents bought this exact house when I was 11 and sold it when I graduated high school almost 20 years ago. There are *so* many wonderful memories I have growing up in this home, in this neighborhood, and with my parents. Now, not only do my children get to create their own memories here, but I get to create new memories with my family here.

Best of all?

There's a room for Mom.

CHAPTER 15:
The Present... It Begins

Continuing April 2021

I may have left out some little details about the backstory of my mother's diagnosis and the events that led to the decision for her to come live with me, but this brings this up to speed into the present where major details come into play.

Biggest update since we found the home we'd been looking for?

We got the house!

We actually get the keys next week. There's plenty of work that has to be done prior to any of us moving in: flooring, widening of doors, installing ramps, etc. Our plan right now—though we all know how plans go—is for us to be moved in by the end of May and to be able to bring Mom home with us at the beginning of June!

The goal is to celebrate her 72nd birthday in the home we will share together.

Her partner is staying where he is, an hour up north in the home they purchased together. He loves my mother, and we love him too! He has done more for her than anyone ever really would have. He has gone above and beyond. They had envisioned a life together once Mom retired, to travel and do things, but her diagnosis pretty much obliterated that dream. It's not anyone's fault. At this point, Mom needs more care than he is physically able to provide, and it would be too dangerous for them both if they ignored that reality.

Right now, I am riddled with a *lot* of questions, concerns, hopes, and dreams. I've been calling around and talking to people I know that deal with home health, hospice, private caregivers, etc. I want to make sure I have everything we might need ready for when she comes.

I want to give her my all, just as she has done for me my entire life.

CHAPTER 16:
We Got the Keys to Our Future!

May 2021

We got the keys to our new home today!

So many mixed emotions happening all at once. We have been searching for our "forever" home to raise our children in since before they were born. I never imagined our "forever" home would be my childhood home that my parents raised me in.

There are a lot of renovations to be done to accommodate my mother's needs, but it should only take a few weeks at the most. Then, we will get all moved in and settled, and if all goes well, Mom will be moving in before her birthday in June.

It's becoming real. I'm excited but also scared, and I'm worried I might be missing an important piece of this very vast puzzle. I'm very good at being one of those "sunshine and rainbows" kind of people who get really excited about an idea or project and forget to ask the important questions or to sit back and *really* think things through. I'm more of a "we will figure it out as we go" type of person. This annoys the hell out of my husband who is a realist and the exact opposite.

I'm keeping faith that I'm not missing anything, though. It's all going to work out. Even with the kinks and roadblocks I know we will face, in the end it will be as wonderful as it is terrible!

Chapter 17:
There Is Just a LOT

May 2021

A. Lot.

The contractors are moving right along with the revamps needed before we move into the new home. This includes new flooring (all hardwood), barn door in the opening from the den to the living room, widening of doorways, installing ramps inside as well as outside, carpeting, etc. It's not a lot, *but it is a lot*.

In the 20 years that happened between the first time I lived here as a child to living here now as an adult, the home had been altered inside drastically with removing of walls, completely changing of flooring, and widening of door frames that weren't the same as before.

It's a lot because of the importance of some of these things to ensure my mom is comfortable and safe. The biggest concern I have is that I want her to be able to continue to take showers. The house she lives in now is very spacious in the bathroom, perfect to utilize the Hoyer to lift her on the shower chair in order for someone to help her shower.

In the house we bought, it's a tight squeeze with some random angles. The main bathroom door was only 28 inches, so they've widened it to 36, but it's the door I'm having trouble visualizing. I really don't care that it'd knock someone's knees off if they're on the toilet because the toilet is behind the door when it opens. That bathroom wasn't like that when I lived here as a child. (Who puts the toilet there? Weird people, that's who.) But I'm trying to visualize how to get the Hoyer lift in there for her to be able to be placed on the shower chair. The shower itself is perfect. Do we use the Hoyer to do it that way? Do we use a sliding/swivel transfer bench? Do we put a rubber mat so she can be wheeled via a shower chair? Is there room for that? Because the vanity is at a disadvantageous angle as well.

All I want is for my mother to be comfortable.

She's leaving a very large home to come live with us. Her room isn't nearly the size she had there. I'm just concerned she's going to feel like she's in a box. Our new home is over 2,000 square feet, so it's not a box by any means, but I'm worried it won't be enough *for her*.

Then, there's the caregiver situation. How the hell do we go about this? I'm going to continue to work full time and I don't want her to be lonely during the day, but I also don't want someone up in her space all day long either. She needs help going to the restroom and laying down for a nap. Lately, she's been needing help with meals and drinks too—prepping for them and even squeezing ketchup or cutting her meat.

My goal is now to figure out how to get someone from about 8am to 5pm, Monday through Friday, who can work with her on transfers, showers, and food preparation. But what do they do the rest of the time!? Mom is going to want some privacy, some space! I suppose I need to stop sitting here, trying to find solutions, and actually make calls and get help figuring it out.

My mind is just overwhelmed.
My mind is excited!
My mind is frustrated.

I am so anxious.

Chapter 18:
Taking a Breath

May 2021

The house is coming along. We've had a few glitches here and there, which is to be expected, but we are on the home-stretch now. We are looking to move ourselves in on Memorial Weekend. Mom had trouble getting movers scheduled, but she was finally able to find someone for the week after July 4th. That puts her moving in about a month past our original goal.

It's just a month.

Unfortunately, with ALS, a month is *everything*. Every moment matters. The kids and I went to see her this past weekend. It'd been about two weeks since I'd been up there and already in those two weeks, major differences could be seen. Her arms are weaker. She isn't able to lift them very high and her grip is diminishing as well.

I am so worried that by the time I get her here, she'll have nothing left of her arms – just like her legs are already. I feel selfish with this thought. I wanted so much to get her home, to get her out and about, to enjoy going out to eat. She won't want to do any of that once she can no longer feed herself. I feel that time is coming soon. I'm not even sure if she'll want to go anywhere once she's completely incapacitated with her arms. I sure hope she does.

ALS is such a monster. She is literally being imprisoned in her body while her mind is completely aware. Again, I'm dealing more with the "not fair" aspect for her and also for myself. It's really been bothering me lately and I'm almost to the point I think I may need some help from my doctor with the rollercoaster of emotions I've been experiencing.

I'm snapping at my kids. I'm depressed about *everything*. Small triggers set me in a whirlwind of emotion. It's not fair for anyone and I absolutely hate it. I tell myself to breathe and relax and then

I'm good for a bit. Until I'm not and it all goes downhill all over again. Once the house is together, that'll help. Getting Mom home and finding that routine, that'll help.

I just want her to be safe, comfortable, and happy. I want to do everything I can for her. I don't want her to suffer. I don't want her to be sad. I don't want her to *leave* me. I'm not ready.

CHAPTER 19:
Crunch Time

June 2021

It's been a bit since I've been able to write because things have just started to happen so quickly but in *such* a good way!

We moved into the house over Memorial Day Weekend. I'm already so much in love with the space, the neighborhood, the memories that were once made and the memories that will be created. To have bought my childhood home just feels right. I can't explain it. I moved into this home the summer before my 5th grade year and lived here until after high school graduation. My daughter is going into the 5th grade this fall, and she's taken up residency in my old room. That's pretty cool, I have to admit.

I do have memories of the home it used to be but only in flashes. We've been here for a week now, and there seems to be more popping up as I roam around the house. We've got so much more work to do, but I'm proud of what we've accomplished in the week we've been here. And by we, I mean my husband. Good Lord, that man is handy and such a hard worker! I'm extremely blessed—that is for sure!

This weekend I am getting Mom's room as ready as I can make it. I'm getting it cleaned, painted, and the furniture I bought her all assembled. She'll come with her hospital bed and her equipment, but I wanted to get it as ready as possible. July 6th is her official move-in day. My siblings and I will go up on Father's Day weekend and start packing her up.

Mom came to visit the house last weekend, and I'm glad she did. We were able to ensure she could move about the house, turn around in the bathroom and bedrooms in her chair, and that the ramps were good. So far, so good! The only problem is that she can't open the doors to get out, especially to the back deck where I know she wants to enjoy coffee in the mornings and bask in the sun during the afternoons. I'm going to try and figure it out for her.

She's got a lot of emotions going on too. Who wouldn't? This is *so* much for her. She's leaving behind a man who loves her but just physically isn't able to take care of her safely anymore. She's leaving behind a beautiful home. She's leaving behind her puppy, Sammy, since it just wouldn't work out at this point with our family dog. She's coming to live with her daughter because she physically cannot take care of herself. Mom is progressing pretty rapidly now with the loss of mobility in her arms and the grip of her hands.

I still have to get the caregiver situation figured out and time is running out on that. I just don't know how to go about it. I want to make sure it's right. Other than that, we are taking it one day at a time. We've got a month before her arrival. Within that time, my daughter is attending three different summer camps, has softball nearly every night of the week, and both my daughter and son have their birthdays and their parties coming up.

Mom's birthday is this coming Sunday. She will be turning 72. Praise be another birthday to celebrate. I pray we have more. We need more time. *I* need more time.

CHAPTER 20

Saying Goodbye and Hello

July 6, 2021

In the midst of all the chaos that has happened between getting the keys to the house, renovating the inside to ensure Mom's mobility is safe, packing all her belongings up, scheduling the movers, and preparing for everything we can for once Mom actually moves in—we unexpectedly lost our 12-year-old Shorkie named Garby.

She had developed symptoms of extreme panting 24/7, and after a trip to the vet, it was determined she was suffering from the later stages of Cushing's Disease. She's probably had it for years and we didn't realize it. Her blood work was off the charts, and her heart and spleen were three times the size they should have been. *That* was one of the hardest days of my life. I took off work and spent time with her while the kids were at camp and my husband was at work. I cried for days and then off and on again for weeks. I still get teary eyed thinking of her. I miss her so much.

There has just been so much heartache for our family lately and this just added to it.

The kids celebrated their birthdays, which are only nine days apart, and this year is the year of separating their parties, as they are too *cool* to have them together anymore. My daughter celebrated her 10th birthday at the end of June, and my son celebrated his 6th birthday at the beginning of July. Both parties consisted of friends, cake, ice cream, presents, candy, and bounce houses.

Although "birthday season" at our house is exhausting, it's over as quickly as it begins, and we don't have to worry about it for a whole year! In between their birthdays, on July 6th, is when we brought Mom home.

But let's back up a few days—primarily Sunday, the 4th of July. It hit me that day that this was the last weekend before Momma was going to be living with us. I was wanting to get all the cleaning and laundry done and grocery shopping completed. I was putting the finishing touches in her room, and I wanted to relax and unwind all at the same time. I knew life as we all knew it was going to change in a monumental way. For all of us.

I was overwhelmed. My anxieties got the better of me for quite a while that weekend. That night, knocking back a few drinks with my husband, I think I went through every single emotion there was. I was excited, scared, angry, confused, lost, happy, worried—you name it and I felt it. At this point we hadn't lined up all of the caregivers. Momma and I were facing a lot of "unknowns" before she even got to us.

My sisters and I went up a few weeks before and packed her up the best we could, so the movers wouldn't have to do so much when they got there. It's a memory I'll never forget, and I'm very thankful for the two of them and the help they brought along. Although I know I'm not alone on this journey, having their help was a nice reminder of that.

After drinking all those feelings down the night of the 4th, we got busy on the day of the 5th and got the house as ready as we could make it. On Tuesday, July 6th, my niece, her girlfriend, and I drove the hour north to Momma's house. When we pulled in the movers were already starting to bring things out. Momma was sitting in her wheelchair in the middle of her living room just watching.

The look on her face was not one that can be defined in just one emotion nor is it an expression I will ever soon forget.

Devastation.
Anger.
Sadness.
Defeat.

I couldn't blame her. I *wouldn't* blame her. This was yet another thing that ALS had taken from her. I was angry *for* her. Once the movers got everything packed, I loaded mom up in her wheelchair van, and my nieces took to my van. As we pulled out of town, heading to her new home, Momma started crying and said, "My life just sucks."

It didn't hurt my feelings. I hurt *for* her, though. Because it does. Her life sucks. Absolutely fucking sucks. ALS has taken so much from her. Although we knew there were rough times ahead, we'd both accepted that this was what had to be done.

Chapter 21:
I Don't Know What the Hell I'm Doing

July 14th, 2021

The first two days of Momma being home have been *the hardest*. Although I have a license to run skilled care/nursing homes, I do not have a license to actually *do* the care. There's a big difference there.

Quickly, I learned I didn't know anything when it came to using the Hoyer lift to safely transfer her from her chair to the bedside potty and back to her bed. Clearly, in planning for logistics and everything else, I simply overlooked the fact that I don't know what the hell I am doing. I was scared. I didn't want to hurt her.

We called a close friend who is a CNA (who will also be one of her caregivers), and I could never thank this woman enough for coming to our aid. For nearly three days she came to help put Momma to bed in the evenings and get her up in the mornings. I watched and I learned until I finally got it. For the first few times of using that lift with her, I sweat so badly that it was rolling off my forehead and dripping onto Momma. But in the week since she came home, I have gone from taking nearly an hour to get her transferred and settled to being able to do it in 20 minutes.

I was off the whole first week she was home. We got a routine down and are still tweaking it here and there. Thankfully we are both creatures of habit. I'm making sure to keep her clean and lotioned, and she's making sure I back off and give her some space! She's still working, because my mother is amazing. After you get her up in the mornings, she's pretty self-sufficient except for transferring, fixing her food, or going to the bathroom. At night, I get up about three times to turn her. She hurts so badly and can't lay in one position too long, and she cannot turn herself.

Now that I've returned to work, we have caregivers coming for the first five hours of the morning to help assist her in all of that.

Then, she sits and watches television, works, or hangs around until the kids and I get home around five o'clock.

We began interviewing caregivers during this first week. The three girls we had come in knew us well, because all three of them had worked as CNA's not only for her, but for me when we both were Nursing Home Administrators. This is something that we have been very blessed to have in our small town—knowledge of people and how well they do their jobs. I could trust them one hundred percent with the care of my mother, no questions about it. In many cases that's not something that is easily available for those searching for caregivers.

Many towns and cities have resources such as lists of private sitters. Reaching out to local Area on Aging organizations is a start. Local hospitals' case management departments perhaps have lists of individuals as well. Reaching out to assisted living, nursing homes, home health, and hospice agencies as many of their CNAs and nurses look to do private sitting on the side. One could even utilize social media. No matter which avenue you take to look for someone to watch a loved one, be sure to get references and get to know them before they begin working for you. We were lucky, considering our experience and years in long-term care in a small community, but that doesn't mean we won't have road bumps along the way either.

I've enjoyed having Mom home. To say I wasn't freaking out this time last week would be a total lie. It's been a complete game changer just making time for one another and getting things done. We are going to have troubles but there's so many more blessings than there are hardships at this point in her progression.

CHAPTER 22:
Finding a Routine in Our New Normal

July 20th, 2021

Funny how in 2020, the phrase "finding a new normal" was coined due to the pandemic. Now in 2021, pandemic-wise, we've gone slightly back to the "old normal." Although, as I write this, positivity rates are skyrocketing yet again here locally.

Now in 2021, my family, and my mom are all adjusting to a different kind of "new normal." Things have been going well thus far. I am getting better at finding a work/life balance, which is now harder than it was last year at this time when the world was smack-dab in the middle of a pandemic, and I was running a nursing home.

The caregivers we have for Mom are phenomenal. I am truly blessed to have these ladies caring for her while I'm at work. In the evenings, after working a long day, is where I've got some work to do. I want to be able to cook dinner, spend time with my family, and get mom ready for bed comfortably (bathing, lotioning, etc.), and I've got about a two-hour time span to do all of that.

Adding in the doctor and eye appointments my kiddos have in order to get them both ready to start school. At this time, we still need to get school supplies and clothes, especially for my son because the kid has shot up over this summer like no other. He doesn't have a single matching pair of pajamas that actually fit.

Tie that in with making sure my relationship with my husband stays fresh, working on house work, and continuing to work on getting Mom settled. I feel like a squirrel running any and every place in all directions at once. There isn't much "down" time, but I know that's coming. I can't tell you the last time I sat and watched a television show, much less a movie. It's not just because Mom's with us—she's just added in along with having small kiddos and a full-time career.

I'm making it. Even on days I feel like it's impossible or I'm failing. I'm making it. They're all alive, well-fed and mostly clothed. That should give me bonus points somewhere, right?

CHAPTER 23:
Mom and the Banana Split

August 2nd, 2021

My goal with Mom is to get her out as much as I can, besides just going to doctor's appointments and such. The past two weekends we've gone somewhere. One day it was to cruise down Main Street and look at all the shops and then we stopped for ice cream. A few things we realized on our journey that day were:

1. It's ridiculous how many stores are not equipped to allow wheelchairs to even enter, much less get around.

2. People *will* stare. Not just kiddos, but grown-ass people *will* stare.

3. A person's best intentions will sometimes get the better of them. Like the lady who made a comment that Mom's chair really goes fast, and Mom simply replied, "I would rather be walking, trust me." To which the woman replied, "Well, you will—you just have to work hard for it." Yikes.

4. Mom's limitations sometimes aren't apparent until it's right there in front of us. Such as the banana split.

Mom loves banana splits. *Loves them.*

We decided after shopping to go get some ice cream, and as we pulled in, she commented, "I haven't had a banana split in so long." So, we got a banana split. Sitting it in front of her, we both turned our heads in question and realized, how the hell was she going to eat this?

Mom no longer has use of her arms from her shoulders to her elbows. She's not able to raise her hands very high, even just to put a spoon to her mouth. At home we have a table that goes over her wheelchair, and we usually prop things with pillows so she's able to get food to her mouth. Here we were, out in public without our table and pillows.

I watched as she tried. *Boy*, did she try! But she was unable to get that spoon in her mouth. We asked the workers if they had a box we could try to put on her lap, but that didn't work. At this moment, Mom was getting frustrated and embarrassed. My heart hurt for her so badly. We ended up throwing it all away (because she absolutely did not want me to feed her there) and got a chocolate milkshake instead.

It's moments like these, that come way more often than they should, that break my heart for my mother.

Chapter 24:
Camp COVID

August 3rd, 2021

We had a vacation planned as a surprise for the kids this summer. We had rented a condo in Florida and were going to take them to see the beach for the first time ever! However, we decided to buy a home, and things just didn't work out on going on vacation. So, the vacation was canceled (thankfully, they had no clue). With a new house and Mom moving in, I wanted to make sure the kiddos were still going to have some kind of adventure this summer; this included sending my daughter to a week-long summer camp in the next town. She was *so* excited!

The first two days without her I was having so much trouble with her being gone. I missed her. I couldn't talk to her. It was driving me insane. Then, two days after we dropped her off, we got a call from the camp. They were shutting down because a counselor had tested positive for COVID.

It gets better: that COVID positive counselor was my daughter's bunk counselor. She had been exposed!

This meant not only was her week of camp cut short, but she was now on the journey of a 14-day quarantine to her room. Thankfully we have a house with more than one bathroom, so she's taken over the hallway one; but other than that, she's permanently in her room. We are now on day 8 of quarantine and so far, so good with no symptoms or anything. She's bummed she's having to miss the first few days of school, but really, she's just tired of being alone.

I mask up and spend time with her. Playing games, watching a movie, and so on. But it was imperative for her to stay away from the rest of the family, but especially Mom. The common cold could kill her because she cannot sneeze or cough due to the ALS. So, no chances can be taken.

Calgon. Take. Me. Away.

CHAPTER 25:
An Itch You Can't Scratch

August 3rd, 2021

Mom started itching. Itching *everywhere*.

It started off completely terrible, and although it's gotten a little better, it's still rough. We have no idea what's been causing it. We thought maybe because we used different laundry detergent than she did, so we switched to hers. That didn't help, so we switched to the dye-free, all-clear stuff. Didn't help. We tried some antifungal ointment, thinking it was fungal maybe. Nope. Her doctors called in some Atarax, and it does help somewhat.

We've been dealing with this for *weeks*. Every night I legit use a hair brush and "brush" her back. It feels *so* good, she says. We started using a loofah for bathing when I noticed dry skin flaking off. Using that has helped a little, but we are still itching.

I went to CVS and bought every single kind of anti-itch cream and lotion. Some help, some don't. *Nothing* totally fixes it. We are still perplexed as to what's causing this. Those in the ALS forums believe it's part of their nerves misfiring, and other PALS (Person with ALS) have experienced it as well. Neurontin seems to help it, they say, but she's already on that. Although we are thinking she maybe needs a higher dose.

It's driving her crazy and I hate it for her. Could you imagine having an itch you can't scratch? Imagine that itch covering your *entire* body.

Finally, with a double dose of both Atarax *and* Benadryl at night, the itching seems to have lessened some. We utilize this along with scrubbing with the loofah during baths and lotioning up and down every single night with Sarna lotion.

CHAPTER 26:
What *Kills* Me Is Seeing Her Trapped Like This

August 3rd, 2021

I don't know how she does it. I guess it's because she doesn't have a choice. This is her life. This is what has been handed to her. It's unfair. Why her?

Mom doesn't question that. She always says, "Why not me?" Sometimes that pisses me off, because she's right and I know it.

Lately we've hit more downs than ups. She's frustrated as she begins to lose more of her mobility with her arms and hands. She doesn't give up though. She'll fidget and fight to get that food to her mouth or a straw to her lips. She maneuvers her notebooks and laptop so she can still continue to work. She does it all, but lately the frustration is evident on her face, in her voice, and in my heart for her.

Knowing this is just going to continue to get drastically worse, I'm finding myself panicking on the inside. When she loses the ability to work, what will keep her occupied during the day while the kids are at school and we are at work? She already cannot let herself outside, though we are looking at a system for that. Eventually, she won't be able to move her arms or hands at all, and even though we are looking into the Eyegaze communication system for her, what kind of life is this?

That's something she says a lot. She says she has nothing to look forward to, nothing to really live for. What kind of life is it to just waste away, she'll ask. This is one of the foremost reasons why she has decided against a feeding tube or ventilator. Why prolong an existence limited to lying in bed, staring upward and not being able to move or, eventually, communicate the way she wants?

HOW DOES SHE LAY THERE AND DEAL WITH THIS!?

It keeps me up at night. I find myself praying for her to be called *home* before it gets drastically worse. Before she loses her voice, her ability to swallow, her ability to express the kind, warm, and wonderful woman she is.

No, it isn't fair.

Why *not* her?!

Because, Mom, you worked to build your whole life from nothing and made it beautiful. No one deserves this disease, but especially not her. Why can't I have my mother grow old and gray as we shop for orthopedic shoes? Sure, maybe she'd need a walker to help get her from point A to point B, but still be walking. I see so many women in their seventies and eighties, and it angers me. Just to see a sweet old lady walking. What's that say about me?

I'm not being selfish. I'm not hurting on the inside because of *me*. My mother has taught me everything I needed to know about life and so much more. I'd be lucky to be half the woman she has been, but I also know my mother and her wishes. I know that once she has taken her final breath, I will be devastated and lost. But I won't live there in dark emotions. Because my mother has taught me resilience.

What kills me is seeing her trapped like this. Seeing her frustrated and sad. It's absolutely heartbreaking.

CHAPTER 27:
Everyone is Busy, I Get It

August 10th, 2021

We are starting to find a routine again. I think it's just always going to be something we adjust as time goes on. Thankfully, my daughter's exposure did not lead to COVID, and she was able to start school just a few days later than everyone else. Our son started Kindergarten, but he had to have the stomach virus the weekend prior to his first day. Everyone had upset stomachs that weekend, including Mom. Nothing like having to rush, rush, rush—something so simple to us is such a big ordeal for her.

Things continue to progress with her. She's starting to lose the ability to move some of her fingers. She isn't sleeping well either. She's up about every sixty to ninety minutes needing to be turned. It just hurts her to lie in one position too long. I have an egg crate mattress coming in today to see if that will allow her to sleep on her back longer since she rests better that way, but it hurts her rear end if she's there too long.

Caregivers have been wonderful, and I would truly be lost without them. I'm worried they may not stick with us for the long haul, but I can't allow myself to stress about the future, especially if there's nothing certain to prepare for. I continue to work full-time while trying to be the best mother, wife, and daughter I can be. The people in my life deserve it. I seriously am so blessed with my family. My husband is patient and kind during all of this. Our kiddos are phenomenal. They truly are amazing. My mother-in-law is connected and helpful and always willing to be there. I have lucked out in the family we have here, and I know not everyone has that.

I talk to my siblings and other family that live locally, but not near as often as I thought I would. They've visited a time or two as well, just not near as often as I thought they would, or as often as I think Mom would like. Everyone is busy—I get it. There are times

I get really angry and frustrated that they said they'd be here so much to take her places and do things with her, and that never has happened. I get angry because it hurts *her*. They don't see that look of hurt or disappointment on her face, but I do.

I don't complain. Unless you ask my husband, then he'll tell you I complain all the time to him. I vent to my husband because we all deserve that one person we can unleash on. Sometimes, we just need to talk it out. That's why I started writing this—not only to record the journey, but also to have a place to let things out. This is a difficult time for my mother. Getting into a new routine has been a challenge for everyone. We expected that going in. I wouldn't change or trade it for the world, though. I wouldn't change or trade it for the world–unless, of course, I could remove ALS from the equation.

I just want to show my appreciation and my love for her. My understanding. I want to be with her, side by side, through this just as she always has been there for every great and difficult aspect of my life. I sure hope my kiddos will do the same for me.

This won't be a forever situation with us. Each day brings us closer to another day gone. I understand that. So, I soak up all the good and laugh with her through the difficulties. Because that's how we are going to survive this. Even though ALS will take her away from me, she's going to go knowing she is loved, respected, admired, and adored.

Chapter 28:
"I Just Want This to Be Over."

August 11, 2021

Those are the words my mother says. She has every right to those wants and feelings. I'm sure many of us would feel that way in her situation. But as a daughter, it hurts me to hear it.

"I want this to be over."

"I don't want to go through with this."

"My life sucks. There's nothing to look forward to."

"I can't do a fucking thing on my own."

"I just wish I'd die tonight."

Those are REAL feelings right there. Strong, true, braised feelings that hit me in the pit of the stomach. Don't be fooled—this isn't about me or how it makes *me* feel. I feel that way because I wish for that too for her.

We don't live in a "Right to Die" or "Death with Dignity" state. I wish people with terminal illnesses such as ALS who are not going to get better could be allowed to choose how they end their own suffering.

Yes. I pray for my mother's life to end.
Peacefully.
Now.
Before ALS takes what little she has left.

I'm not a monster. It's what *she* wants, and I want it because she wants it. That doesn't make me a monster. That makes me sincere, compassionate.

Fuck ALS.
That's it.
I just want to cry.

She doesn't want to be fed. She just refuses. I support her refusal of a feeding tube 100%. But she's having trouble getting food to her mouth now and won't allow me or anyone else to help. She said, "I won't be fed. I won't allow it. Just let me starve to death."

We bring up hospice during these feelings but she's not wanting that at this time. She's frustrated. I'm frustrated. We are fixers and neither one of us can fix this.

Fuck ALS.

It needed repeating.

CHAPTER 29:
Two Pink Lines = One Panic Attack

August 17th, 2021

My daughter tested positive for COVID today.

We learned Thursday she was exposed by a friend on Wednesday. She went back into quarantine (this poor child) *again*. On Sunday she began to develop symptoms: fevers, headache, body aches, and slight cough. She didn't feel terrible, just not well. Went ahead and tested her and she tested negative. Having worked through the pandemic last year, I know it's possible to test too early.

Yesterday, she had a fever, and her coughing had gotten a bit more frequent. Still, she felt okay. She hadn't been eating as she doesn't have much of an appetite and says some things don't taste right.

Today she had no fever, just a cough. We went ahead and tested her so that she could return to school. Positive. Awesome.

Also, today I woke up with symptoms. My head is "full" and hurts, my throat hurts, and my chest is tight (I'm asthmatic). I tested negative but I know how that can go so I will be testing again Thursday.

I kept my son home with us yesterday and today just in case. Glad I did. Now my daughter is in quarantine until the 24th, and my son is in quarantine until the 30th. So far, he doesn't have symptoms, but if I test positive then he has no hope. The kid is always right next to me.

The adults in the house are vaccinated. So hopefully if we do get it, it'll be mild. But even mild COVID can be detrimental to Mom. ALS has taken away the ability of her to cough or sneeze.

I'm worried. Hell, worrying doesn't even cover it.

My daughter has been in her room since Friday. Today when I started feeling off, I began masking around my mother while I care for her. Could be too little too late.

This is a lot.
Just—a lot.

CHAPTER 30:
Today is Another Hard Day

August 27th, 2021

Thankfully no one else ended up with COVID, but nothing else is going right for Mom. Her body is continuing to fail her, and she becomes desperately frustrated with herself and her circumstances. I don't know how to help most of the time, which aggravates her even more. I knew as the ALS progressed that she would become depressed, angry, and frustrated. Who wouldn't? I knew that with me being her caregiver, that anger would turn towards me a lot because I'm the one constant here. Knowing that and going through it are two *very* different things. It hurts, but it hurts differently than you'd think. It hurts because I cannot help her or control her circumstances any more than she can. I hate this for her. *Hate it.* As her body declines, everything becomes even harder.

She's leaning to her right as she's in her wheelchair now. Her trunk muscles are going. She is completely paralyzed from her shoulders to her elbows, and now the forearm muscles are going as well. Her hands and fingers are failing. It won't be long until she is a paraplegic. I'm not sure where we will go from there.

She is still working (she's amazing, *I know*) on her computer as a consultant, but those tasks take SO much out of her. She can't type so she uses a pen and taps on the screen. Getting things set up and within reach becomes more difficult every single day. And that's just for work. Eating continues to be an issue. She's swallowing okay, although she has choked a time or two. We have the suction machine ready and the cough assist device that works as a motorized suctioning machine through a mask, though I have no idea how to use it yet either. She cannot lift her utensils to her mouth, and now finger foods are becoming harder too. We have her set up with a bedside table over her, a contoured pillow around her, and other pillows to prop and lean on. All of which worked for a bit. All of which are now failing.

She refuses to be fed. I think I covered that earlier.

So where do we go from here?

She's tired so often and will lie down to take naps, which has been okay since I've been home the past two weeks from work (because my daughter was COVID positive, and my son had to quarantine due to that). I believe my mom was hoping she would have contracted COVID and that'd be that. She said, "It'd be easier than to go the way I'm going now."

I worry about returning to work next week. Our caregivers are here from about 8:00 in the morning until noon. Mom was able to manage by herself from noon till about 5 p.m. when I got home. But in the last two weeks, she's needed much more assistance during that time in having to use the restroom or be laid down. Do I get caregivers for the afternoon? That could be hard to find. Do I quit my job and do my duty as a daughter? Financially, mentally, and emotionally, I don't believe that's the answer.

I don't think anyone knows the answer.

At night, she's up every hour needing to be turned. When she moved in, it was about two to three times a night. Now it's about six to eight times, depending on when she goes to bed. When she's turned on her side, she's not able to stay there long, as her body won't allow it. I have wedge pillows to try to keep her on her side, but they hurt her shoulders (she has terrible arthritis in them). Everything seems to be working against her. Everything is working against me.

This wasn't how I had imagined it would be. Don't get me wrong, I knew this time would come, but it came so fast. I thought we'd be out running around town, going out to eat, friends and family visiting. I imagined us sitting on the back deck with our coffee, watching movies, and enjoying our time together. Instead, we have skipped right past most of that and into depression and frustration. If she gets to the point, and she will sooner rather than later, that she can't work, then I don't know what is next. She'll watch TV for quite a long time (she's rediscovered the show *ER* and binge watching), but she can't do that all the time. Can she?

No one comes. She's had visitors, but not as many as she and I had expected. I am thankful for those who have taken the time to see her, but I'm disheartened at the absence of others. Yes, I know everyone is busy, and really this past month, we've been on COVID precautions left and right. I get that, but we have family in this area that has yet to see her. We have some family that's seen her once. We have some family members who proclaim on Facebook how she's their everything, and before we moved her in, they told me they'd be here. I've yet to see them.

I know that sounds terrible. I'm not bitching for myself. I take care of her and don't expect anyone else to. It's not the caretaking. It's socialization. She's getting sick of me, I am sure! You just really see true colors, you know? I should say more to them, but I don't want them to visit out of guilt. I just don't want to hear their shoulda-coulda-wouldas on the day Mom is gone and they no longer have the chance.

I do miss sleeping full nights.
I do miss going out to eat with my family.
I do miss having date nights with my husband.

It's also important to know that I would have made the same decision of bringing her home.

I'm allowed to have bad days.
I'm allowed to feel frustrated.
I don't show or tell her about them.

CHAPTER 31:
Vehicle's Don't Bounce Off Curbs

August 28th, 2021

After weeks of quarantine, we wanted to get out today. Mom had an eye appointment to get her glasses for the Eyegaze communication system. It's a computer that allows you to work it with just the movement of your eyes. They're for those who are paralyzed. It's very interesting! They're coming on Tuesday for that.

I was excited. We got up early and got her in *actual* clothes, not just pajamas. Her hair was looking good, she was smelling good, had her makeup on and everything. Five minutes before we were supposed to leave, she says she has to get a certain paper for the doctor.

We couldn't find it. Anywhere.

That set off the mood. No more good morning. Things were flying, she was frustrated and yelling. I was in tears. She finally found what she needed, and we went to the eye doctor. Late, but we made it. Tensions were so high. Sometimes it's hard to get her out of the funk once she's there. The eye appointment went okay though, and by the time we left to go to the farmers market she was better.

We actually got quite a few things at the market. It wasn't too hot yet and it was just nice to get out. The wheelchair still doubles as a great bag carrier. At this point in the day, we both apologized for the morning. We were back on our way to having a good day.

It didn't last very long.

Another stop was the pharmacy. Upon leaving the parking lot, I took a curb too sharp and wrecked the passenger side of her van. Badly. It jarred the door that housed the ramp slightly open and crushed the body mechanics of it. We were able to drive home with alarms sounding.

My husband and I were able to get her out of the other side of the van using an emergency ramp we had, but now the van is totally out of commission. Thankfully, we got her eye appointment and blood work done today. We've got someone coming on Monday to look at the van to see where we go from here.

Upon arriving home, Mom had to quickly use the restroom, although there is no such thing as *quickly,* with as far as she has progressed. Mom is leaning terribly to the right. She doesn't know if it's her chair or her body. It's her body. You can't position her comfortably anymore. Which hurts her and frustrates her. And the moods continue.

I'm unraveling. I'm trying not to, but I am.

Chapter 32:
This Is All a Temporary Strife for a Lifetime of Gratitude

September 1st, 2021

Mom can no longer brush her own teeth. She can no longer wipe her own face because her arms are going fast. She's been nauseated for a few days and today got sick. Dizzy. Blood pressure was fine. COVID test negative. It's just been a day.

Today, my mother put in her 30-day notice for the consultant work she's been doing. The one thing that has kept her going was her work. She has become weaker as more of her body continues to fail her. She cannot do it anymore, and it's breaking her heart, which means it's breaking mine too. I work my eight hours every day knowing she's sitting at home with just a television to entertain her and it's gutting me.

Thankfully she has agreed for us to get caregivers for the afternoon now as well. The day caregiver will do 8:30 a.m. till 1:00 p.m., and then we will have someone else from 1:00 p.m. till 5:00 p.m. (when I can get home). Caregivers can start having her go outside to the porch or on the back deck to sit when it's not so hot. They'll be able to take her for a ride or to get lab work (when the damn van gets fixed). At least she will not be alone. The caregivers may be bored, but they're there in case Mom needs something.

Just this past weekend, my daughter and I had to rush back from Walmart because Mom called crying. Her arms had dropped to the outside of her wheelchair, and she didn't have the strength to lift them back up anymore. The people for her Eyegaze system were supposed to have showed yesterday but didn't. After waiting an hour past the time they were supposed to be there, we called and were told they didn't have enough help to come down and forgot to call us. Great. I wasted a day off for that. So, it has been rescheduled for later this month, along with her trip to Indianapolis to the ALS Clinic.

We are going to have to look at getting her chair adjusted because she isn't comfortable anymore in it. She's leaning too much, and her bottom is getting sore. Her hands can't reach the controls and her arms won't stay on. We also need to look at a few medication adjustments as well. She has a dentist appointment, hair appointment, Eye Gaze appointment, ALS specialist appointment, and it's all *this* month. My son also has a dentist appointment this month. My daughter has both an orthotic appointment and physical therapy appointments this month. I'm also supposed to get a root canal (I've put it off three times) next week. Seriously, I don't see that happening. My daughter auditioned and got a part in the local middle school musical (she's in elementary school, just a handful of younger kids got in!), so rehearsals will start for that.

I don't want to take anything away from my kiddos. I want them to be able to get to their appointments and practices and rehearsals. I want to do crafts and play with them. I'm starting to slip down the "way too much going on" slope, and I need to hit the brakes. I need to take a deep breath and organize my thoughts and my life. Time management is key here.

I can do this.
I'm doing this.
I'll continue to do this.

Because my hero, my mother—that's what she's taught me. She is going through hell right now. She did not want this life for her or her family, but it's what we've been handed, and we are going through this together. She saw me crying this past weekend. I usually am good at hiding it from her. I get frustrated with the situation, not with her, but she thinks it's the opposite.

At the beginning of her diagnosis, we often prayed for slow progression so she'd plateau and save what she could. We don't pray for that anymore. She doesn't want to live this way any longer than she has to. She knows what's coming. We both do. All we can do is take it day by day and pray that she does not suffer and that we can make her comfortable—not only physically, but mentally and emotionally as well.

CHAPTER 33:
We Had to Call 9-1-1 for the First Time

September 11, 2021

I had come home from an elementary school PTO meeting and was getting Mom ready to go to bed. She had been complaining about headaches for days, and tonight was no different. Except, when I was about to put her in the Hoyer lift, she looked at me and said, "Cassie, I'm going to pass out."

Suddenly, her face was flushed, and she started to hyperventilate. I grabbed the pulse ox, and her pulse was racing at 176. She began crying and saying her arms were numb. I immediately grabbed my phone and called for an ambulance. The next few minutes was her crying as I watched her heart race. My daughter was in the shower, but my son was right there. He was such a good helper. He went and grabbed both our purses and her glasses as I manually guided her chair to the den.

The firemen arrived before the ambulance and did her vitals. Her heart rate went from 176 to 58 and back up again. I watched as her oxygen levels plummeted. They put her on O2, which I later learned was the wrong call. ALS patients can't exhale the CO2, and it can cause confusion and disorientation, which it did. I had known that but forgot it all in the chaos and worry.

The ambulance arrived and they loaded her up. That was terrible. Her arthritis was so painful, and she cried out. She was in and out and kept repeating, "I am a DNR!" I remained calm. I kept telling her I loved her and was right there. In my mind, I wondered if this was it. I wasn't allowed in the ambulance, so I ran to my car and went to the ER.

When she got there, she was a bit better but was so very confused. I later found out this was because of the oxygen they had given her. Thankfully, she didn't need it anymore. Her pulse was improving, and so was her blood pressure. They did a CT, chest X-ray, blood work and EKG. Everything turned out okay, except that her potassium was low at 2.7. She takes supplements, and we'd been working to get it up. Just the week before, it had been 3.6. Not sure what happened, but it seems like low potassium could have been the culprit of this episode.

They discharged her, but we had to get IV potassium first and then wait for an ambulance to bring her home, which was around 4am. It was such a long and uncomfortable night for her. All I wanted was to get her home and comfortable in her bed.

She slept most the next day. I reached out to her doctors and specialists. I also tried to sleep but didn't have much success. Yesterday was a much better day for her, and today she's great. Her headaches aren't so bad and she's back to herself quite a bit.

It was scary, but all in all we were calm and prepared.

I had a dream yesterday that she got up and walked. I found out later she also had the same dream. Creepy. I believe in signs, and it makes me wonder if we both know she will be free of this horrible disease soon, because we both know she will walk again when she's in Heaven.

Chapter 34:
My Heart is Breaking

September 18th

I put her to bed crying.

I can still hear her through the monitor.

"I don't want to live like this, Cassie."

I never know what to say other than:

"I know, Momma."

CHAPTER 35:
Taking Myself a Break

September 19th, 2021

This past weekend was Homecoming in our small town. When I tell you nobody does Homecoming like my town, I mean it. This year was my 20-year high school reunion. For months, I planned to ensure it could be done.

I had doubts.

Our village pulled together. My husband got us a hotel room for two nights. My sister came and stayed all weekend, learning how to do the Hoyer lift and how to turn mom at night. My mother-in-law watched my kiddos. We had two caregivers come to assist mom to bed and to get her up in the mornings.

I had moments of guilt for not being home and helping. I was reminded it was okay. Funny, I used to say the same thing to families when I would market the respite care programs of the nursing facilities I worked in. It's different when it's *you* going through it.

It was a wonderful weekend filled with fun, comradery, and too many drinks. I owe so much to our village that made it possible.

Mom spent most of her weekend parked in front of the TV binge-watching ER. She likes the show and watches it a lot. Her work for her nursing homes is slowing down. She only has two weeks left—the end of quite an era. It's bittersweet.

Actually, for her, it's just bitter.

So much has been taken away from her. So much. It isn't fair to see her this way. Sad, depressed, frustrated. Heartbroken.

I wish I could do more for her. Her van is still in the shop, so she hasn't been able to leave the house in two weeks (except for the darn ER).

She wants to give up. I know she does, and I don't blame her.

I have never hurt so much for someone as much as I hurt for my momma.

CHAPTER 36:
The Love of Family

September 20th, 2021

My daughter wrote an essay for school. It was about what makes her happy. She wrote about her grandma living with us. She wrote about helping rub lotion on her, helping prepare her meals, and getting things to her since she can't do it for herself.

My 6-year-old son scratches her back, adjusts her feet, gets her pillows right, and this past weekend, he helped her eat some chips.

If anything positive comes from this journey, it's knowing I am instilling in my children the love of family. They will remember these times, and although some have been scary and more will be sad, I pray they remember the good they did for their grandmother. I hope they know how much good they did for me too.

CHAPTER 37:
Another ER Trip

October 5th, 2021

We've had quite a hectic few weeks at our home, starting with the explanation of Mom going to the Emergency Room *again*.

One afternoon while I was at work, I got a frantic call from one of the caregivers. She fell off the ramp! She had been going down, and she couldn't lift her fingers off the joystick and kept it going right. And up and over the ramp she went in her power chair. I raced home, as the caregiver had called 911. Seeing Momma lying there, trapped by the power chair and crying, made my heart skip a few beats. The rescue workers were able to get her out and onto the ambulance to get to the ER.

The caregiver had literally thrown herself at Mom to help cushion the fall, which in turn bruised the heck out of the caregiver. The power chair's seat belt saved my mom, because she ended up without anything broken or even bruised!

Needless to say, we've ordered a new ramp (wider and sturdier), and it's arriving today.

This past weekend (right after the accident), Momma got to have a weekend she had been looking forward to: her sisters (all four of them) came to visit from Kentucky!

It was pure chaos at the house, but the good food, the laughter, and the memories created made it all worthwhile. I wish they lived closer so Momma could see them more often. She's wanting to go down there to visit, but we are *still* waiting for her van to be fixed from when I hit the curb over a month ago. We should have it back next week, hopefully, as she needs to go to the doctor, the salon, and the dentist. It'd be nice to get her out of the house some more.

I am constantly worried about her depression and state of mind. She's no longer working, so she just gets up, has breakfast, and watches TV all day long. I don't know what to do to keep her a bit more entertained, because by the time I get home, she is constantly feeling like she is a burden to me (and she most definitely is *not*). With nicer weather, we hope to take some strolls around the neighborhood at least, and once we get her van back, we will go places, even if it's just to look at things.

I don't want her quality of life to suffer.

CHAPTER 38:
Adding Eight Paws

October 6th, 2021

We have officially lost our minds. We. Are. Insane.

We welcomed Lucy and Molly as the newest members of our household. They are miniature labradoodles. We brought them home two weeks ago.

They are adorable. They are smart. They are *a lot*. They are chewing everything (including each other) and making messes all throughout the house. As much hard work as they are creating for us all, they are also good puppies. Most of the time, if they make a mess inside, it's in the den on a puppy pad. They nap like champs and usually sleep well through the night. My husband may have to get up once with them.

The kids love them. Absolutely love them. There was no rhyme or reason to why we got them when we did, other than that we wanted to fill an empty void in our hearts. We miss our Garby so badly, and we knew it'd be best to get them while the weather is good (for potty training purposes) rather than when it's cold and snowy outside.

The kids aren't the only ones who love them.

They have brought Momma smiles and entertainment. They sometimes will lay on her lap (Molly, who is smaller, especially) but she's been so good at keeping an eye on them. Her caregivers look after them during the day, which is *super* helpful.

So, I guess we aren't completely insane.

Just, you know, moderately insane!

CHAPTER 39:
ALS Is the Gift That Just Keeps on Giving

November 10th, 2021

Mom's needs are forever changing. What works one day doesn't necessarily work the next. You have to be able to think on your feet at a moment's notice because her comfort and safety are at risk. The newest item on the "that's weird" list is sticky hands. Yes, sticky hands. The other day mom said her hands needed washing because she must have gotten syrup on them somehow when I was feeding her waffles. The woman loves her waffles. I felt her hands, and sure enough, they were sticky.

Not like a normal sticky feeling. It was as if she had dipped her hands in glue. Her fingers were sticking together, and my hands would stick as I held hers. We used hot soap and water. No improvement. We used a wipe. Nothing. Her hands would have been able to help her scale the side of a building—they were *that* sticky. She said she'd noticed it a few times before, but every night I put lotion on her, and I had never noticed. I wouldn't have, though, because I had used lotion. Lotion! I grabbed a hold of her favorite Bath and Body Works lotion and rubbed it on her hands. The sticky went away.

Since then, she's had it happen a few other times, and lotion is the only thing that keeps the stickiness at bay. I had gone to my ALS Caregiver support group on Facebook, and sure enough, others have had this issue. They had recommendations such as baby powder and apple cider vinegar, but what worked for us was lotion.

This goes along with her itchy skin I had posted about before. That's still an issue, but it's not as terrible, so long as I continue to do our nightly "scratchings." I use a loofah and scrub hard all over her areas that itch, which is about 90% of her body. Then, I take an anti-itch lotion, usually Serna, but Gold Bond (the mint green one) works too. I rub her down with that. Then, she takes 50 mgs of Atarax. It doesn't solve the issue, but it does give her some relief.

Again, what works today very well may not work tomorrow.

CHAPTER 40:
Struggling to Find the Balance

November 10th, 2021

It's been going on five months since Mom came home to live with us. I won't lie—some days it feels a lot longer. It's taken us this long to really start learning to find a balance. Usually when I start feeling like I've got a routine down, (I am a creature of habit) something finds a way to kink it. I've been striving to be the best daughter and caregiver to my mom, but I lost sight that I also am still a mother and a wife. Also, I am a person myself.

In the last month or so, I've made it a point to have some family fun. With Mom's van still in the shop (this shipping crisis the country is in is for the birds), Mom hasn't been able to attend some of the things we've done as a family, but that is okay. I've learned to say that is okay and that we can still go out as a family of four (husband and the two kiddos) and just BE us. We've taken the kids to Holiday World, we have had a lot of autumn fun with Halloween and pumpkin patches, and we even made it on live TV when we attended WWE Smackdown Live (husband's choice, obviously).

I arranged for caregivers to be with my mom so that we could do all of this. I used to feel guilty for even leaving Mom to go to Walmart, but it's what she wants. She wants me to still be me and do things without her and be with my husband and family. It's taken me a bit to understand that this actually makes her happy to see and hear all about it.

I had these visions of what it would be like when my mom moved in. Going out to eat and shop all the time. Her in the kitchen telling me how to make her recipes. Family and friends coming in and out of the house to visit. The reality is, with ALS or any terminal degenerative disease, expectations are rarely met. Mom's progression was in full swing by the time she came to live with us. Where she used to be able to sit up and type on her laptop and scroll through Facebook on her phone, she is now completely paralyzed with minimal movement of her arms and hands. She can't hold a tater tot, much less her phone.

She didn't like getting out because people would stare. It really irritated me when people would speak to me about her when she was *right* there. I wanted so much for my mom's quality of life to be more than just getting out to go to the doctor. When we crashed her van, her freedom out of the house halted.

She gets up, she's fed breakfast, and she sits in front of the TV and watches her medical dramas. She's already watched the entire series of ER and is just about done with Grey's Anatomy. She's fed lunch, she lays down. She gets up, she's fed supper, and she goes to bed. In between, we talk about our day and other things, but she essentially goes from point A to point B and back again.

So even with her van in the shop, I found a place that rents wheelchair vans and will be getting one for this weekend. She's going to go see my daughter in her musical. She's going to go to Walmart and take a stroll along the riverside. Gawkers be damned— she's going to get some fresh air.

As important as it is to spend time with my family unit, this includes her 100%. My son loves to do family drawings, and I've noticed in the last month or so, when he does this, he always draws his grandma, wheelchair and all.

Tell me our children aren't watching us. Tell me their childhood experiences don't shape their future.

CHAPTER 41:
Certain Rewards Make Hard Things Well Worthwhile.

November 19th, 2021

This past weekend was my daughter's musical. She loves the performing arts and was cast as part of the ensemble during the local middle school play, despite still being in elementary. Mom had seen her a few summers ago in their production of *The Jungle Book* and again two winters ago in *Elf: the Musical*, but she'd missed the last few for various reasons.

She wasn't going to miss this one, especially now that she lives here! Mom's van is *still* in the shop (don't get me started), so we had to make a drastic call. We got in touch with a place about an hour south of us that rents out wheelchair accessible vans. It was well worth the money and the drive to be able to get a vehicle for Mom to be able to get out of the house. It's been months since we wrecked her van, and she's been cooped up inside this entire time.

We first went to Kohls, just me and Mom, to do some shopping for winter clothes and a new coat. For the past few months, Mom has only had to use her wheelchair to come out of the room, up the ramp, and park it in the living room—then back down again at the end of the day. So, going shopping made us realize, yet again, just how much ALS has taken from her.

She cannot lift her left arm anymore, but she does have a few fingers that work. We lift her hand onto her lap, and she can use those fingers. She can slightly lift her right arm (not well), but her fingers on that hand are contracting and losing muscle. She can barely use the joystick to her wheelchair anymore. She doesn't have the strength to keep it going or use her fingers to wrap around it. We had to stop—go, stop—go, stop—go. This was fine for me, but I could tell it bothered her.

It was the same that night at the musical. It was super cold, very windy, and having to go from the wheelchair parking spot to the school's door was brutal. She did it, though. My Momma never gave up, and she just kept going. She got to see the musical. It wasn't so much even seeing Mom's face during the performance that impacted me as it was to see my daughter's face light up when she saw her sitting out there.

Certain rewards make hard things well worthwhile.

We have decided it's time for me and Mom's daytime weekday caregivers to learn how to operate her chair from behind with the controls. It's for Mom's safety more than anything. She hates it. It puts a damper on her mood, but she also knows she's surrounded by people who won't give up making sure she has everything she needs.

I got an email from the body shop that her van should be ready soon. We aren't going to let anything stop us—failing grip, failing muscles, cold or wind—none of it. We're going to get out of the house as much as we can once we get that van back.

CHAPTER 42:
Perspective.

November 20th, 2021

They come out of nowhere sometimes. In the middle of the day, watching television, a thought crosses her mind. Just an instant of a passing thought, and tears fill her eyes.

"I don't want to be this way anymore."

"I don't know why I keep holding on."

It's in those moments that I know better than to pacify her with a silver lining because there are no silver linings with ALS. At 72 years old, my mother has dedicated her life to others. Raising her sisters. Working to put herself through school. Raising her children. Taking care of my father for 10 years after his cancer diagnosis. When the moment came for her to focus on *her* life, ALS came, halting any prospects of traveling and enjoying her "golden years."

She would be the first to tell you that she doesn't question, "Why me?" Because she always says, "Why *not* me?" However, as her daughter, I am constantly questioning, "Why her?"

To see her body fail her daily. To see the pain (physical and emotional) roll through her eyes. I want nothing more than for her to be free. My mother is my best friend. My confidant. My role model. My heart. My world will be so dim without her physically on this earth.

I know.

I know it's selfish to want that. To ask her to fight. I am doing my best to keep her as comfortable as I can, to give her everything I have, and I wish upon everything in the world that it hadn't been her. Her advice to me growing up—through hardships at school, a failing past marriage, and hitting rock bottom—was always, "Suck it up and deal."

That's what she's doing. She shouldn't have to. I couldn't, but I am nowhere near as strong as her. I don't have half her resilience and dignity. I'm a big-ass baby.

But for her, I'm sucking it up and I'm dealing. What I feel isn't even an ounce of what she's feeling.

Chapter 43:
Inflatable Bathtub, Who Would Have Thought?

January 2nd, 2022

All Mom wanted was a shower. When she first moved in, we thought, "We can do that." We quickly realized we'd underestimated how much her ALS had progressed, even in July. There was no way she'd be safe to sit on a shower bench, even with a gait belt strapping her to a chair, for a shower. It was disheartening for her, and it broke my heart to see that for her.

For months, we did bed baths. The caregivers are really good at giving them (I'm not the best, but I try), but it still wasn't like soaking in a hot tub of water. Mom's body becomes contracted, and her muscles ache all the time. She had bought an inflatable bath tub last year, having known the need for it would eventually come, and a few of the caregivers decided to try it out.

It is *such* a cool system! They lay it out on her bed and inflate it. It looks just like a kid's inflatable pool. Then, they place her inside it (while it's dry) and take her clothes off. The hose runs from the sink in the bathroom next door and starts to fill while she lies there. There's an inflatable pillow inside there as well. They let her soak in warm water for as long as she wants, and when she's done, the hose then becomes a drain and drains back into the sink. They rinse as it drains and then dry her off, lift her up, and deflate the tub before placing her back on the bed (after putting sheets back on it) to get her dressed.

They've done it a few times now, and she's loved it! It takes about an hour and a half from start to finish, but it's totally worth it.

CHAPTER 44:
Looking Back on 2021

January 3rd, 2022

So much has changed in so many areas of my life.

* I left the nursing home after 18 years and embarked on a new position and new career with our local hospital (best decision ever).

* We sold our home of 12 years and moved into my childhood home (gained a bedroom, a den, larger kitchen, yard, deck, and two more bathrooms).

* Our furbaby of 12 years, Garby, left us to go to Heaven.

* We added two new furbabies, Lucy and Molly, and that's been an adventure.

* My daughter started her last year of elementary school and will be in Middle School in 2022.

* My son started kindergarten and has had some struggles with behaviors that have caused an increase in my production of graying hair.

* Momma moved in with us (biggest thing to happen in 2021)!

Thanksgiving was a grand gesture of over 30 people at our house (my side of the family). It was great to have everyone together, but it was overwhelming for both my mom and for me. We planned Christmas a little differently, and it went well. We had some come on Friday, some on Saturday, and then some on Sunday. That enabled Mom to actually visit with the ones who came, which was nice for her.

Since Thanksgiving, things with Mom's ALS have started to progress *even more*. The most concerning is the contracting of both of her hands. Her caregivers and I massage and try to prop them open, but her fingers are curling, and her hands ache all the time.

We've noticed she's leaning more, and we've got the guy coming out soon to start more adjustments on her chair.

Most recently, her eyes have started to water and mat quite often. We wash them out morning and night, but we're having to wipe her eyes a lot because she cannot do it for herself. It's the same when she has a runny nose. She can't lift her arms or straighten her fingers to blow her nose, so someone has to do it for her. That's become very frustrating for Mom.

Other areas we've noticed are her memory, especially short-term. She's becoming more forgetful and "spacey" which, after this last ALS Clinic a few weeks ago, we've learned it's probably her CO2 rising in her body. She's never been one to want to use her Trilogy machine (non-invasive ventilator), but she now knows she needs to. She gets out of breath if she talks for too long. We've got respiratory therapists coming to show me how to clean the Trilogy (because it's dusty) and how to properly use it, and then add on the mouthpiece for her wheelchair for her to take a "quick breath" when needed.

The good news is that we *finally* got Mom's van back after being in the body shop for months. So, she was able to get out a few weeks ago and go see her new doctor and get a flu shot. I want to be able to take her out more and do some shopping, but it's so cold as I type this. We are all learning how to control her chair as she cannot do it herself anymore, not even just a little bit. She's lost that much of her hands and wrists. So, we take her everywhere by using the controls for her chair. They're not as easy as you'd think, but we are learning.

Christmas was bittersweet. Maybe it's because it was the end of the year, the end of an exhausting holiday season, or just because we knew what it was–our last Christmas with Mom. We aren't being morbid, just realistic. I'm glad to have had her with us. She enjoyed watching the kids open their gifts and seeing them play with their new toys. Depression is hard anytime of the year, but the holidays make it worse, and Mom was no exception. Her mortality is something she speaks of often:

"I won't be here for this next year," or "I just rather be gone than sit here and watch everyone else's life pass them by."

It's hard. On everyone.

It's not harder on anyone more than her though.

We are about to try some new medication to help with her pain management. I'm working hard to try and make sure she's got nutrition, because her appetite has gone and she's starting to choke a little more each time. We are all doing the best we can, including her. There are hard days, but there's also just as much laughter as there are tears. For myself, I intend to work harder in writing (New Years Resolution Number 48,290,485).

Here's to making 2022 the best we possibly can!

CHAPTER 45:
We're Starting the New Year, and Things Are Crazier Than Ever

January 4th, 2022

Around 2 a.m. I was awoken by the disgusting sounds of my husband being sick. I was selfish at first in my thoughts of, "Now I'm going to have to take out the dogs, deal with work, the kids, and trash day, on top of a sick man, which is worse than a child." But my tune changed quickly when I realized my husband had a 104 fever. Yikes.

I quickly got up and took care of the dogs and the trash. Got the kids ready for school and dropped them off. Hurried to CVS for a rapid COVID test and ran home. He was negative. I quickly did a conference call, emails, and some reports before getting said husband to the doctor. They did a PCR COVID test as his symptoms are all lined up for it, the flu was negative. Could it be a belly bug? Guess we will find out tomorrow. He's still currently sick as a dog with a very high fever.

I burned through some more emails, another conference call, and then went to get him his meds. Shortly after I came home, Mom wanted to be "bent over" in her chair. Sometimes that relieves pressure on her bottom. However, this time she went into a coughing spell, (she's got a cold, which is scary for ALS warriors) and she turned blue as she couldn't get her breath!

It took a few moments that seemed to last forever before she got a good inhale of oxygen. Did I mention the respiratory person was coming today to set up her new equipment, but we canceled due to sickness? Smooth move, right?

She's better now, though she has a headache, and I'm just staring at her. Thankfully, a caregiver was here with me, and we both stayed calm as she struggled for her air. That hasn't happened before. This is new. Could it be the cold? She can barely cough due to her diaphragm being affected by the ALS. This is our future, we know, but is it already here?

She doesn't want a vent or PEG tube. I'm honoring her wishes, but this reality just slammed itself into me a few moments ago.

This is going to happen, and it's going to happen sooner than any of us would ever want.

Now it's time to get the kids from school, take the dogs out, make supper, do homework and showers, make sure the hubby is surviving, and get Mom ready like I do every night for her bedtime routine.

Maybe I'll take a shower tonight.
Maybe I'll have a glass of wine.
Maybe a glass of wine while in the shower.

This is *fine*. We are all fine here.

CHAPTER 46:
Momma Went Viral!

January 7th, 2022

I belong to a Caregiver support group on Facebook for ALS Warriors and their caregivers. We trade ideas, seek advice, and vent to one another from time to time. I've gotten a lot of great ideas from them, and I've helped answer some questions as well.

I thought it'd be a great idea to share the inflatable bathtub system we used for Mom. It was great for her, and she really enjoyed it, so I figured others may want to look into something like that for themselves or the person they care for.

I had no idea it would blow up the way it has on Facebook! As of today, the post has been shared over 33,000 times! All over the world!

At first, I was super stoked that it had been shared over a thousand times. I thought, "Wow, that's great!" This post was made three days ago and I'm still in shock every time I check Facebook and see more shares. I love reading the comments, answering any questions they have, and seeing them tag so many people in it for ideas for their care.

The best part is the huge smile Mom gets when I tell her how much it's grown. She loves that others might get to enjoy a nice hot soak, something many give up on when they reach the condition Mom is currently in. That's the best part.

Despite how much she has declined, she's still giving.
She is still inspiring.
She is still making a difference.

CHAPTER 47:
It's Getting Worse as Each Day Goes By

January 8th, 2022

We know this is part of the progression. Not every ALS Warrior is the same. ALS progresses differently for nearly every single individual. However, my mom seems to fit the textbook Sporadic Limb Onset ALS diagnosis.

When her symptoms first began (late 2018/early 2019,) it started with her uneven gait. She wobbled. It then moved to her feet, which caused her to trip and fall. This was summer of 2019. By the autumn, she was having to physically lift her legs in and out of the vehicle. From there, it moved upward. Both legs nearly simultaneously. She was 100% wheelchair bound by early 2020. It then moved to her arms, and we entered a period of slow progression, almost a plateau. By early 2021, she was losing her arms, not able to lift them as high. By summer of that year, her arms from shoulders to elbows were essentially nonfunctional, and her torso (trunk) was incapacitated to the point that she could no longer sit on the side of the bed.

The progression accelerated, and that was when she moved in with us. Her elbows to her wrists went next, and she only had her fingers. By December, she no longer had the use of any of her fingers or her wrists. Her hands started to contract, which was (and still is) painful.

Now here we are, the beginning of 2022. She's had a few instances where pills she swallowed would get stuck in her throat. Then at times, food would be slow to go down. Now, it's more often than ever, for both pills and food. She hasn't yet choked on liquids, but that'll come too.

Tonight, I made one of her favorite meals: fried pork chops, fried potatoes, and butter corn. We have tried slowing down, smaller bites, chewing better, and tucking her head down as she swallows.

I'm not sure if she just was really enjoying the meal and didn't chew enough, or if we were going faster than we should, or if this is just yet another sign of progression, but she choked. She choked *big time*.

I don't panic. I'm a person that always stays calm in emergencies. When she has swallowing issues, I always just stand still, watch, and listen. I make sure she's either coughing a little or there's air moving. Usually, there is. Tonight, there was a moment during this spell that I heard a whistling breath and knew it was going down the wrong "pipe."

This is especially dangerous due to the fear of aspiration. I've seen it a million times in my field, but it hits differently when it's your mother. It took a moment, but she cleared it without us having to scramble for the suction or cough assist.

It's coming.

One of her wishes is to not have a feeding tube. We've already agreed that when it becomes too dangerous, then she's "just done." We still have a ways to go. We can alter the texture of the meals (as much as she doesn't want to), but I'm hoping she will change her mind. Just like she did with being fed. She swore she'd never let anyone feed her, but for months now, that's been the only way she can eat, and she's grown accustomed to it.

I'm always going to honor what she wants. Tonight, just set another stone of reality in this ALS journey of ours.

Chapter 48:
I Do It All with a Smile on My Face

January 10th, 2022

I'm lucky I have a husband who picks up where I slack off when it comes to laundry, dishes, and floors. When I get home from work and the caregiver goes home, I "clock in" as my mother's caregiver. My husband doesn't get home until a few hours after me, so I get the kids from school. We come home, take out the dogs, and I immediately start supper. And let's face it, it's usually something simple these days.

As soon as the caregiver goes home, it's my spotlight. Mom isn't able to move. Now that it's winter, everything is itching her everywhere. It's also part of the ALS. We lather with lotion and scrub her to get dead skin off. She takes medicine for itching. Yet, she still itches. Now, her scalp is itching like crazy too.

On top of that, ALS has also caused hair loss. She's constantly having little hairs fall down onto her cheeks and nose, which drives her crazy. Who wouldn't be driven mad with that? With all of this!? Not even being able to wipe off a hair or scratch your arm. Let's also throw in that when she's got a cold, (she's just getting over one) and her nose is runny, she can't wipe it.

The point to this is—what she can't do, I do for her. I am her hands and her feet. I wipe away the hair. I scratch what itches. I wipe her nose. This is usually all worse in the evenings. So, while I'm cooking said simple dinner, trying to rein in the kids, and take away whatever the dogs have gotten into, I'm also at her beck and call for all of the above.

It's part of what caregivers do, and I know sometimes when my husband is walking past with laundry in his hand as I sit in a chair next to my mom, he's had fleeting thoughts of "she's doing nothing." At least, that's how I feel: guilty. I should be doing chores

113

too. He doesn't say things like that though. He knows. He hears it and sees it too.

Don't get me wrong, I still do housework, but in the evenings I'm Mom's hands and fingers. It wouldn't serve any purpose for me to move at the moment because as soon as I do, she calls out. She usually calls out the moment I sit down too. She's also notorious for calling out about 10 minutes before my alarm goes off in the mornings.

She apologizes sometimes, and I worry I've had a frustrated look on my face or let out an audible exacerbated sigh. I don't mean to. I'm human. Just like she can't help it, sometimes I can't either.

I'm not ranting. I'm just marking the routine to show myself that, as much as I feel like I am not enough as a daughter, a wife, a mother, a friend, I know that I'm doing what I can. I do it all with a smile on my face, in front of my mother at least.

CHAPTER 49:
Mom Has Been Sleeping More

January 20th, 2022

We use the monitor when she's asleep so I can hear her call out for me.

I'd like to say she's resting more at night, and that's true to some extent. What's different now is that she's napping much more during the day. Sometimes (like today) she's up for about an hour and a half to two hours and then goes back to lay down for a good three hours (sometimes more). She gets up for a little while and then goes back to bed at night.

There have been many nights I've been up to turn her every hour. Lately, there's been some longer stretches, which is good for us both. However, she's calling out for me in her sleep without realizing it at times, or she calls out "Mom" or one of her sisters' names. There are times I go in there and she doesn't remember what she wanted or forgets I had just been in there the last few minutes. Sometimes she tells me to turn her to her back when she's already laying on her back.

The confusion is there during the day as well. She's repeating herself a lot. I've noticed she becomes quieter though too. I know these signs because I've worked with these signs. She doesn't talk as much because she's confused. I'm sure her CO_2 is up, which causes the weird dreams, the napping, and the confusion. She's trying the Trilogy machine again but just for an hour or so during the day until she can get used to it more. The goal is for her to wear it at night so that she rests more and isn't as tired during the day.

I'm not looking too far into what this may mean, but those of us in healthcare know. It's an omen just as much as it's a progression of her disease. Mom hurts a lot, especially in her bottom, back, arms, hands, and wrists. We can no longer turn her without causing her pain, and I hate that more than anything. The way I have her in bed at night is almost comical to us now. With as many wedges and pillows, splints, and supports as it takes to ensure she's as comfortable as she can be.

ALS is a monster.
Simple.
Period.

CHAPTER 50:
Particular Bed Time Routine

January 21st, 2022

There's a certain way my mother has to be placed in bed at night.

Her "wings" are towels to prop up the sides of her pillow so she can turn her head left and right and still feel the pillow for her cheek to rest upon. Her head is the only thing she can move now.

We laid a pillowcase over her chest for her hands to lay on so that her fingers don't snag in the buttoning of her pajamas, and then the hand splints for her contractures.

A small wedge at her bottom helps alleviate pressure from her coccyx area.

A folded blanket elevates her heels. We have tried numerous things for her heels. This is the best so far but still not perfect. We can't do anything high or it hurts her legs.

When I turn her to her side, it's much simpler. All that comes off, and we have another wedge that goes in the back to help keep her in place and a pillow for her arm to rest on so that shoulder doesn't hurt.

We rotate about every two to three hours. Although, some nights she can't get comfortable and it's every hour or more.

Send coffee.

CHAPTER 51:
I Am Getting *So Sick* of My Own Name

January 28th, 2022

It literally makes me *cringe*.

This is because it's constantly being called. My momma can't help it, I know. I'm her hands. If she can't scratch her nose, blow or pick it, if her eyes are running, if something needs to be moved or scratched, then it's me. If she hears the dogs or a noise, she's calling my name to ask what's going on, what are they doing, where are they? It's me.

It's a lot.

At night she calls when she needs me to turn her, to turn her heated blanket up or down, if she needs to use the bathroom, if she needs a drink. And sometimes she doesn't remember why she called out to me. Sometimes she says it in her sleep. Sometimes I hear it in my sleep.

When I get home from work and I'm trying to wrangle the kids, the dogs, supper, housework, I'm interrupted constantly by all of those above along with Mom calling out my name to do something.

I'm not bitching—I'm just ranting because it is *a lot*. I know one day I'll miss her voice. I'll miss her needing me. Just like I'll miss the kids being little and fighting every five minutes.

Right now?
This very moment?

I'm gritting my teeth as I await the next "Cassie." The thought makes me grit my teeth and seriously contemplate changing my name.

CHAPTER 52:
Extra! Extra!

February 9th, 2022

Read ALL about - My Momma!

A local magazine did a feature on my mother, the love she gave teaching young CNAs and Nurses, and how that love has come around in *her* time of need. The five girls that take care of her while I am at work once worked under her and are now returning that love.

I'm pictured on the cover with all of my mother's caregivers surrounding her. I never think of myself as a caregiver. I'm a daughter who takes care of her mother.

The story was written with such love. The author truly captured my Mom's story and did so with such talent that it'll be something my family cherishes forever. It encapsulated the essence of my mother who spent a lifetime leading charge to take care of others family members. She did this with love, dignity, and high expectations that all of her nursing home residents would be treated like family. Mom treated her staff like family as well. She is an educator by passion, and this is a virtue that continues with her to this very day.

My favorite part the author wrote was:

"For life has dealt one of the world's most beautiful one of its most debilitating blows."

So very, very true.

CHAPTER 53:
There Are Moments That Make Me Stop

February 10th, 2022

Sometimes there are points during this journey that make me pause, suck in a breath, and swallow the lump that's formed in my throat.

Last night was one of those moments. As I was taking Mom to her room, she started to cry out of nowhere. She wouldn't tell me why. Our whole bedtime routine was punctuated by her crying silent tears and me gently brushing them off her cheek.

I hated it. She hated it.

I gave her a hug and kiss before I left her to sleep. The exchange between us was silent but the meaning that hung in the air was screaming.

Today she had a doctor's appointment to get a cortisone shot in her shoulder. While talking to the orthopedic doctor, who is friendly and has a great bedside manner, she suddenly started talking to him about "being done" with it all.

I could see it in her eyes.

The doctor was great with her, and on our way home, she told me that last night she had just felt defeated. Worthless. No purpose.

I told her she has a purpose with me and with more others than she could ever imagine. My mom is a doer. Always has been. To lose the ability to do anything has taken far more of her actual being than I can describe.

I'm going to offer her the opportunity to talk to someone. Alone. Just them and her so she has someone other than just me to talk with. I'll respect her wishes if she declines, but I'm really hoping she says yes.

Talking is good for the soul, and there are just some things you can't or don't want to talk about with those closest to you. I understand that.

Fuck ALS.

CHAPTER 54:
Just One More Thing After Another

February 28th, 2022

If I'm ever lucky enough to catch a daytime weekend nap, I'm often found doing so on the couch with the baby monitor clutched in my hand near my head. This happened this past Saturday and my daughter took a photo of me. Mom had a restless Friday night, which meant I had one too. The old saying, "sleep when the baby sleeps," now means, "nap when Momma naps" if you can. I'm holding the monitor so I can hear if she calls out. Whenever Mom is in bed, that monitor doesn't leave my side. At night, it's right by my head.

That picture my daughter took made my heart feel heavy when she showed it to me. I should have been playing with her and her brother. I should have been cleaning the bathrooms. I should have been doing a lot of things. I was just too exhausted.

As Mom declines, her needs are very frequent. She cannot help it. It's terrible for her. She'd be upset if she ever thought I was exhausted because of her. She sees it. She sees when my name is being called in a million directions either from her, the kids, or our puppies. She sometimes doesn't realize that as soon as I take care of her needs and move on to start or finish another task, she's calling me right back. She doesn't remember.

Mom has been more uncomfortable lately. Her neck muscles are weakening, and she can't hold her head up very well. She can't toss her head back like she used to when she takes her pills. I should also mention her wheelchair is broken down. Something is either wrong with the battery or the charge port, but it won't turn on. It's been that way for a week.

Thankfully, we can still use the chair and just push the 410-pound machine manually. She can't go up the ramp to the living room, where she likes to sit and look out, but we have the den by her room so she can watch tv when she's in there. Since there's no power to the chair, we cannot tilt it back. Her neck has been hurting more because she has to use what little strength she has to hold it up. The vendors for her wheelchair are supposed to come out in a few weeks. That was the earliest they had available. She may have to have a rental if they can't fix it that day.

My kids, especially my son, are expressing their frustration that I never play with them or do anything with them. "All you do is take care of Grandma." Or cook. Or clean. They're not wrong. The moment I get home from work, it's me. From the moment I park on Friday afternoons until I leave for work again Monday, I'm here at the house taking care of my Mom. I am not upset in the least bit; it's what I have to do. I've got to start thinking of ways to help me. Perhaps I could have a caregiver come on two Saturdays a month during the day so I can go and be with my family. My husband and I had a date night the other week, and a caregiver came to put Mom to bed. It was really nice to get out and have a meal. The kids' spring break is coming up, so I thought about using some time off work to do things with them. I get so torn between so many people that I end up losing complete sight of myself.

I went to the doctor today, and I've gained so much weight. I stress eat. I stress eat at work and at night. So, lifestyle change it is. I'll want to exercise and maybe do that when everyone is in bed, because what little time I do have I don't want to take it away from the kids.

I feel guilty for feeling stressed. Isn't that weird? I'm grateful to be on this journey with my mom. It isn't easy, not in the least bit. Admitting that I also need a break shouldn't make me feel like a rotten human being.

Yet, it does.

CHAPTER 55:
Making Our Journey Public

March 5th, 2022

Mom's oldest granddaughter came to visit from out of state today with her family. Mom actually wanted to go for a stroll around the neighborhood!

It was *so* great to get her out into the fresh air. It was a beautiful day, and I honestly think the Vitamin D did her some good. I'm hoping this is the start of her wanting to get out more!

I made my writing public yesterday. That was a huge deal for me because of how personal I get with my thoughts and emotions. Mom knows I'm writing about this journey, but I've only read a few posts to her. Obviously, none of those that I tell of my stress because she doesn't need to hear that.

My hope in this writing is for me, personally, to look back on, but also to perhaps reach others that are caregivers with some advice. Even just letting them know they aren't alone in their thoughts and struggles. This is their journey, yes–but it is *our* journey as caregivers too.

I've already had some readers reach out, and it's a breath of fresh air. Having a loved one depend on you is terrible for them and hard for you. I wish this on no one. However, it's a relief to know we are not alone and to have that support system means everything.

CHAPTER 56:
You Have to Laugh

March 8th, 2022

We have to laugh when we can. Mom is losing control of her neck muscles, so when I have her in the Hoyer, her head is hitting the bar and/or going through it.

Tonight, I wasn't prepared for that and just grabbed the closest thing I could to cushion her head–her fuzzy house slipper!

If you don't laugh through this journey, you simply won't make it. Take humor in the little things. It's the little things that will help to dull the blow of the big things that are out of your control.

CHAPTER 57:
Swallowing a Bitter Pill

March 18th, 2022

This week was my kiddos' spring break. We've yet to ever do a vacation. My daughter is dying to go to Florida. I keep saying "next year," and then things happen. COVID for the past few years and this year, Mom moving in happened. To find someone to stay at my house for 24 hours while we are gone is impossible, especially because of the two dogs as well. I've painted myself into a corner there.

I still took off half the week and I spent every moment of it with them. We did so much, including a day trip to a zoo that's about an hour away. We got to feed the giraffes, which was awesome for me because they're my favorite animal.

They enjoyed themselves and I did too. Now it's Friday, and looking at the weekend, I suddenly get down. Mom has had an increase in depression. I don't blame her. She is frustrated she can't do anything with what she has and is dwelling on all she has lost. I got her to sit outside on the front porch for a while, but she ended up crying, making me take her back inside. You can hear the highway from our house, and she said it made her sad to hear people coming and going when she can't. I've offered to take her places, but she doesn't want to. I try to offer different foods, but she has no appetite and nothing sounds good.

I talked to her about what I've done with the kids the past few days, and she got down and said, "I just sat here." She used to enjoy hearing about the things we'd done together. Now she gets easily frustrated at me and my kids. She often snaps at me when I'm doing her care. I know it's not personal, but it's hard not to take it that way. She's lonely, but half the time she doesn't want to see anyone.

Then, I get down because I get frustrated. Frustrated because no one is here to help in the sense of feeding her or even just talking to her. It's on me to make sure she's engaged, her emails are read, her bills are done. And the hardest is making sure she doesn't slip further into depression. That's all on me when it comes to the family, and it gets to me. I wish it didn't.

I had such a different vision of having others here, wanting to spend time with her while they could, and I'm left with *such* disappointment. I know others have lives, but so do I. I have two small kids, a husband, my career, and myself. I would make the same decision again as to taking care of my mother, but others have no idea what it takes.

The hardship. The heartbreak.

The good news is that I finally started taking something to help with my nerves. My stress was out of this world. It does help. I've even started to lose weight because I'm not stress-eating. I don't admonish others for not coming around as much as they said they would, but I also won't hold their hands when the day comes and they no longer have the chance.

That sounds bitter.

I don't mean to be bitter. I am venting because I have to get it out before I explode. I just take Mom's misfortune to heart, and I put her happiness all on my own shoulders. I know I cannot change her circumstances, but a part of me will always feel as if I am not doing enough.

My kids, though—they really did have such a good time!

CHAPTER 58:
Mom's Body Continues to Fail Her

April 6th, 2022

Recently, her neck has been failing. She's not able to turn it much at all. Her head hangs because it hurts to keep it up. So, of course like we always do, we find a way. A neck collar does the trick. Does she like it? Like is a strong word. Does it do what she needs it to? Yes.

Lately, pain has started again in her legs and arms, even though she has no movement there. She says it throbs like a toothache. We have changed her pain medication, but it doesn't always help. Her back hurts too, and she's leaning more. I believe her spine is no longer holding her upright.

With this comes the long nights once again. Last night, I got *one* hour of sleep. I hated it for her, because she's the one in pain and uncomfortable. Yes, I'm tired, but I can function. As long as she hopefully sleeps better tonight. I'm human, and eventually I'll collapse if I don't rest.

Recently, we had the flu in our house. The kids had to stay home from school, caregivers had to call off, either because they were sick or their kids were sick—or honestly, I was home so they could take the time off. It made for four *very* long days with me and Mom.

I don't like the word "needy." I think it's rude. She requires not just a lot, but almost constant attention. Whether it is to adjust even a centimeter, wipe her eyes that continually water, her nose that's running, or scratch various itches. She's also extremely frustrated and pissed off (who can blame her), and I get the brunt of it.

That's what I am here for. That's why I knew I could be the one to care for her, because I know she's pissed at her disease, not me. As much as I can cry and be frustrated because what I am doing isn't helping her or I do it wrong by her standards, I know it's not personal. That doesn't mean it doesn't hurt.

Mom's mind is also going. I am not sure if it's because of her CO_2 being high or if we are dealing with some dementia. She's very forgetful, becomes very confused, and it's the worst part so far. She gets upset when I try to give her meds, telling me I already did that. She gets mad when I don't put her face cream on, even though I had just done it. She will tell me to hand her something, when she can't move her arms/hands/fingers. She states she just moved in when she has been here almost a year. She yells that we forgot to do her taxes when we completed them weeks ago together.

I keep track of her meds and refill needs, her appointments and things needed for those. I make sure her bills and the caregivers are paid, balancing her checkbook. She has lost all independence, and I hate it for her. She is constantly arguing with my son (who is a handful himself) and in true mother form, she comments on my parenting. That part sucks, not going to lie.

We went recently to get her set up for a new communication device that will allow her to use eye movement to not only control her wheelchair, but be able to get back on Facebook. She misses her socialization. On her terms, though. She says she wants visitors, but by the time they come, she doesn't want them to or she just wants a few minutes and not hours.

Recently, my brother-in-law and his family traveled to our home and put a concert on for Mom. Oh, how she *loved* that! It was such a positive day.

This week is busy with her appointments, kid appointments, dog appointments, and even appointments for myself to prepare for this awesome fundraiser I'm a part of for our local United Way. The first ever Big Balloon Build in the USA is going on here in our small town. It's exciting! Over 125,000 balloons in the theme of Candy Land.

Friday night is a benefit dinner and fashion show. I was asked to be one of the models and I'm thrilled! I get to walk in a handmade dress made out of balloons with my hair and makeup all fancy. This week, I've gotten my nails done, a spray tan, and I get to have professionals do me up before the event. It's something I'm so excited to be a part of, and because of a great support system with my mother in law and our caregivers, I'm actually able to do it.

My daughter has a follow-up appointment at the children's hospital Friday that her dad's having to take her to, as well as auditions for her for a speaking part in this summer's musical. It's busy but I'm managing. So far—it's only Wednesday though.

We're just taking it one day at a time and sometimes one hour at a time.

Once again, it's a temporary strife for a lifetime of gratitude.

Chapter 59

Life Continues to Happen: Good & Bad

April 14th, 2022

My older brother got his photo in the local news. Well, a mugshot of my brother made the local news. That's his umpteenth mugshot.

I start this off with a disclaimer that, just like you and your family, we are by *no means* perfect. This writing is true, and that includes the ugly truth.

My older brother battles with addiction. He has for most of my life. Addiction is a terrible disease that rips away the true character of a person and turns them into someone you no longer recognize. I have very fond memories of my brother, including playing with me as a child, teaching me to ride my bike, teaching me to drive, and always having my back as I had his. There are eight of us siblings, me being the youngest, and this is the sibling I've always been closest to growing up.

Even through the thick cloud of his addiction, I see the true person my brother is. He has been arrested many times, in jail and work release and back again. This time though, he made news headlines, like *actual* news. He made such grave errors that could have—but thankfully didn't—killed not only himself but others.

When he is locked up, my mother and I have always breathed a sigh of relief. Why? As anyone who has loved someone who battles addiction knows, when he is locked away, he is safe. We know where he is. He has shelter. He has food. And usually, he dries out long enough that we sometimes we get a glimpse of the man we know.

This time is different because of the stage Mom is in.

When the news broke and we saw this, her words were: "I will never see him again."

She's not wrong. It's extremely possible he will still be in the system the day she is relieved of all her pain. This, seeing her son once again losing his battle—it kills her. It creates even more pain than her own battle she is losing with ALS.

Last night as she slept, she was dreaming and talking. All I heard her say, or rather groan, was my brother's name over and over again.

That gutted me.

CHAPTER 60:
Happy HallowEaster!

April 17th, 2022

For Mom, it's been a sleepy Easter. She's been having so much trouble sleeping that we finally reached out to her neurologist, who prescribed her Trazodone to take at night.

Well.

She really didn't rest any better—I got up four times with her—but what we have noticed is the "hangover" effect it has the next day. She can barely keep her eyes open. She stayed up long enough to eat but quickly had me put her back down.

But not before telling my mother-in-law, who was here for dinner, *"Happy Halloween."* Yikes. We won't be taking *that* medicine again, that's for sure.

That's what you have to do, keep trying until you find something that works. Right now, we haven't found it, and that makes for super long nights and days, for the both of us.

The kids had a great Easter weekend with coloring eggs, baskets, and an egg hunt, followed by what I have to say was a great meal prepared by me!

Even if you are tired, you have to keep moving on.

Happy Easter!!!

CHAPTER 61:
We Are Coming up on a Year

April 18th, 2022

A year ago, we made the decision to bring Mom home to live with us. I feel like little pieces of myself constantly get torn away, and I never truly heal. I am needed and wanted in so many different directions. I have so much to do, but when I have time to actually *do* it, (for example, cleaning the house), I find myself just sitting and staring into space. Before I know it, an hour or so has passed by and I'm being called by someone again.

As Mom progresses, she's needing more and more attention. I already didn't have as much as I would want to give to my kids, now it's becoming less. And my marriage? Well, less and less do I have the mentality or energy to not only keep up with my motherly instincts, but I feel like my husband and I are just reacting to everyday life. Same routine. Hardly any talking. I know that's normal, especially during times like this. And again, it's only temporary.

I get angry—jealous, really. My husband can do what he wants, when he wants to, and that's pretty much how it goes. He can work in the yard for hours or watch tv and actually sit down for more than five minutes at a time. He has *all* the time in the world to be with the kids.

I end up resenting him because he doesn't really speak to my mother. He just goes about his day as if she doesn't exist. I'm not even sure if that's the truth or if I'm just veiled by my own feelings at this point. I don't know what I expected from him. I wish he'd help to adjust her here and there, ask her if she needs or wants anything, instead of having her completely out of his sight and just waiting for her to, you know, no longer be here.

I'm sure that's just me and not the truth. But it's my truth at this very moment. Life is hard and I'm struggling, but I know my mother is struggling more. My kids are struggling. Hell, maybe even my husband is. We are all struggling, but this is what we agreed on and what we know is the right thing to do, and we want to do it. I just need to learn to control my resentful thoughts and work on positivity more. Maybe then it'll catch on more with my husband and our kids.

This is a lot, more than I can even convey in words. This past weekend, a very close friend of mine shared that she is going through a very scary situation. It's still processing in my mind. Things can change and shift at any moment of any day. You look back on everything and wonder—was it enough? Did I focus on the right things, or did I spend too much time on the wrong things?

It's never enough. *I'm* never enough. To others or to myself. How would that be if I received the same news my friend had? I don't want to wait until it's detrimental for me to change or shift my focus. I should do that now while things are still good in my life. There's absolutely no reason to be miserable or stuck in negative mud.

This was a bunch of rambling.

I feel better.

CHAPTER 62:
I Am on Alert

April 19th, 2022

With ALS progression, sometimes it happens overnight and sometimes it's slow, and at times you even seem to hit a plateau and stop declining.

When Mom started to lose her balance and ended up paralyzed in her legs, it was a slow progression. Years. She plateaued for a while. When her arms started to go, it was faster. She suddenly couldn't lift them at a certain height and eventually not at all. Her hands were quicker. That was almost an overnight ordeal.

For the most part, ever since she's been paralyzed from her neck down, it's been slower physically. Because there wasn't much more mass to be gone. Then her neck started to lose function, and we are still dealing with that, a little more each week.

What had started as a slow progression in her mentality has now begun to accelerate. I wrote about her taking the Trazodone to help her sleep. It did not work. We tried it twice and we were done. She was so sleepy and out of it yesterday, and we believe it was due to the med.

Today she was worse than yesterday. She was up just an hour before she had to lay back down. She was falling asleep as I was putting her on the toilet and then when talking on the phone. She slept all day. She got up for a few hours, and then back down she went. I had her tested for a UTI because lately her bladder seems "sleepy," meaning she can't always pee when she feels she needs to, but the results were negative. If she's still dazed out tomorrow, then I for sure know it wasn't the one pill she took three days ago.

It's a progression.

Her CO2 is rising, and as that continues, she will be exhausted, her breathing will be shallow, and she will be very disoriented. Just like she's been the last two days.

I'm on alert. Something inside of me is telling me this isn't going to get better. Obviously.

Again, fuck ALS.

Chapter 63:
"When I'm Gone..."

April 24th, 2022

Mom has had this Trilogy machine for well over a year. It's a non-invasive ventilator. Kind of like a CPAP/BIPAP on steroids. Because ALS affects the diaphragm, she cannot expel the CO_2 fully when she exhales. This causes CO_2 to back up inside her body. Symptoms of high CO_2 levels are restlessness, confusion, headache, fatigue, and delirium.

Mom is experiencing all of these.

She's tried many times to get used to the machine. Different masks and settings. With the humidifier. Without the humidifier. She's tried to wear it during the day to get used to it so she can wear it at night. She never wears it long. It makes her nose run and eyes water. She says it gives her a headache. She says it's uncomfortable.

Finally, the other night she confided in me. We were getting ready for bed, and she looked over at the machine and started to cry. She said the machine gives her much more anxiety than she can handle. The fact that if she wanted it off, she can't just reach up and take it off. I can understand this anxiety—I have to be knocked out for dental procedures and drugged to get MRI's.

"I just don't want to do it."

That was that. I told her she didn't have to. There's nowhere in the rule book that states she has to do anything. So, we are done with trying it. It's her decision and I will always fully respect it.

Not using this machine means she will continue to decline mentally. She knows this. Her worry is that she will become "hateful" toward me in a confused state. I laughed. I told her she's actually quite pleasant when she's confused!

Since the decision to not use the Trilogy, Mom has really been adamant on making sure her affairs are in order. I have access and know where everything is, and she's constantly reminding me of her wishes. That's our nightly talk as I'm giving care to her while putting her to bed. "When I'm gone..." That's usually how it begins.

Mom keeps talking about my father. He will have been gone 10 years this October. She speaks how he's "peeking" through the gates at her. She smiles when she talks about him. She misses him and has since he left. I know he's waiting for her and she's ready to be with him once again.

Thoughts and conversations such as these are not uncomfortable for me. I am at peace knowing my mother will not be with me much longer. She's in pain. She's tormented with her failed body. ALS has taken everything from her, and the day she is released, I will celebrate her freedom.

I will be heartbroken. I will be angry at how this has happened and taken my mother from me. But I will relax in my grief knowing she's no longer suffering. I will not *live* in my grief. I will feel it, I will express it, but I will take the pain and push forward. Because that is what she taught me my whole life.

"Suck it up and deal."

Chapter 64:
I Am Tired

April 26th, 2022

Emotionally.
Physically.
Financially.
Mentally.
Tired.

I just want to scream.
I honestly feel as if no one would hear me, or even care why.

You're told to make sure you have self-care. But the mention of doing said self-care instantly makes you feel selfish. Or others make you feel selfish.

It's exhausting trying to make a plan for self-care.
And expensive.

I'm just blowing off steam. It's to the top and eventually will dissipate, and I'll start the rainbows and sunshine all over.

But right now, I feel lost. Alone. Depressed. Worthless.

I feel like life is just flying by and I'm not able or allowed to enjoy it.

This makes me frustrated. Sad. Terrified.
Tired.
I feel so tired.

Chapter 65:
Happy Birthday, Momma

June 6th, 2022

Today is Mom's 73rd birthday! We honestly didn't think we'd make it, but she continues to be a warrior.

As I was putting her to bed last night, she made the comment, "Wasn't your dad 73 when he died?" I corrected her by stating he was *almost* 74, and let's not go making 73 that magical Heaven number! She laughed.

This past weekend she was visited by her three of her four sisters, her life-partner, and her brother-in-law. It was a short visit, but it did her heart so good to see them all!

She's been getting a lot of birthday wishes on social media and some videos of people telling her happy birthday. She loved it so much! Another one of my brothers came to visit with her, she talked on the phone to many people, and tonight I grilled her favorite ribeye with baked potato and sweet corn.

My daughter has been away all last week at a church camp, came home for just the weekend, and left again this morning for 4-H camp for a few days. I've missed her a ton, but I know she's having such a great summer so far. Last night after everyone was in bed, she wanted to make Mamaw her favorite lemon cake. Even though my daughter wouldn't be here to enjoy it, she wanted to do that for her. Then today, my son realized she got to bake for Mamaw, so he wanted to as well.

The week before my daughter left for church camp, both the kiddos were in a musical, *Frozen Jr.*, through the local theater camp. My daughter's done it many times, but this was my son's first camp and performance! They both did so great! Mom wasn't able to make it to see it. She's been going to bed by 7pm most evenings, but we recorded their biggest parts for her to see.

Since summer is here, one of Mom's favorite things to do is to go sit outside in the sun on the back deck. The heat feels *so* good on her. She's always cold, which is part of her ALS. She's always wrapped up like a teddy bear with her PJs and electric blankets. But if she gets out in the sun, she's so comfortable soaking up those rays.

Mom's progression at this point has slowed. She still chokes randomly and has pain in her hands a lot. We've got a routine down, but sometimes it's still a lot. I'm constantly pulled in many directions all at once, but I feel I've been managing well. I wouldn't know what I'd do with myself if I wasn't needed by someone, or multiple someones, all day and night long.

Mom still hasn't been sleeping too well. She's just not comfortable most of the time. So, sleep deprivation hits more often than it used to. I know I pushed myself when simple sinus issues went on too long for me, and I ended up with infection in my sinuses, ears, and bronchitis. Currently, I don't have much of a voice, but steroids and antibiotics have really helped me feel so much better.

Oh, I did do something for myself. Call it a midlife crisis since I'll be turning 40 this winter, but I pierced my nose!

Turning 40 is different for a lot of women. I didn't think it would be for me, but it is. I'm not where I thought I'd be in life. In many aspects I'm farther ahead, but in other aspects I'm still falling short of my expectations. A work-in-progress. That's had a whole new meaning lately.

One of my dear best friends found out she has breast cancer that has metastasized to her lungs and liver. This has made me gasp in the air and hold on tight. I've known others, some currently battling, but this person is very close and very special to me. She's also my age. We've been friends for nearly 25 years. We are family. She's just starting her battle, her journey. And even though my plate is full, there is always room for her on it. She's going to fight, and I'm going to be right beside her.

Meanwhile, I'm still keeping my head above water. It's been nice getting into a routine again, but we all know that doesn't last. Things happen, and what works today won't work tomorrow. We, as in my husband and kids, have plans this summer to go on a few short day trips and overnight, so the stress of finding someone to be with Mom all night comes again.

I have a conference in Florida coming up in November, and I'm already stressing on planning that, along with kids birthday parties this month. Alas, one step at a time. That's how we get through it. We do what we can, when we can. And if we can't? Then we don't.

Hopefully, I can keep up with writing more often. It really does help me to get it out and then to look back. We've officially been in our new home a year now, and we are just a month away from the anniversary of when Mom moved in.

What a journey this has been and continues to be!

CHAPTER 66:
Mom's Plateauing Has Come to an End

June 19th, 2022

Her neck muscles are becoming increasingly flaccid to the point that she can barely lift her head up. It hangs down. When she's in her chair we tilt her back so it rests naturally, but when I'm putting her on the Hoyer and transferring her, it just hangs. This is becoming an issue when she takes her medication, because I'd been pouring the pills into her mouth with a cup. She'd take a drink of water and kind of "flick" her head back. That's no longer an option, and now I tilt her back in her chair to take the meds and brush her teeth.

What's got me writing tonight, though, is the alarming new change in her breathing. She actually said for the first time ever last night that she felt as if she were having trouble breathing. She can't take big breaths anymore, and last night catching her breath was an issue.

I then realized that for the last four days or so, she'd asked for some pain reliever for her headaches. She just did it a moment ago. At first, I thought it was the weather, because it's been incredibly humid lately. Although, she's constantly wrapped up in her electric blanket, even when it's over 100 outside. Now I'm starting to think those headaches are because of her lack of oxygen.

As I sit here and listen to her through the monitor, I'm a bit more alarmed. She's doing more gasping than usual. Not deep gasps, but short ones. I wouldn't call it air hunger, because it isn't constant. Maybe air hunger doesn't have to be constant, though?

She has decided against using the noninvasive trach, the Trilogy machine she had. The company even came and got it. There's nothing to alleviate this. ALS has started to freeze her diaphragm. It's progression, and it's end-stage progression. I know this.

The head issue really bothers me. She has a collar we bought to help keep her head up, and as much as she doesn't like it, we are headed to having to use that. I know a lot of ALS patients end up bed bound completely because their neck goes and it's the last muscle she has any control over. I cannot even imagine the terror of only being able to move your eyes. I just can't! Being paralyzed from the neck down has been enough turmoil as it is for her.

That's ALS, though. This monster of a disease will take every single thing you can do away. Right down to being able to breathe.

I've got a feeling.

I know what this feeling is. I'm trusting in my instincts that have always somehow given me preparation, almost like a warning signal. I feel it.

Chapter 67:
Mom Guilt

June 20th, 2022

Mom moved into our home last year when the kids were just turning 6 and 10. Soon, they'll both be having another birthday. That's one full year of their life changing as well.

There have been many times the "Mom Guilt" was thick. I was always the one that would be taking them everywhere and anywhere. I would do games and crafts all the time! When Mom moved in, my attention was split between the kiddos and her. Especially at the beginning, it was more her as we navigated this new journey together.

We are still finding balance and routines, but it is *so* much better than it was a year ago. I often worried my kids would act out or even resent having to share me so much, not being able to go away and do things like their friends were doing.

Then today, picking them up at summer camp after work, I left a little bit early to take them to their favorite store and a quick trip for ice cream before we made it home in time for the caregiver to leave. On the way to the store, out of nowhere, my son spoke up and said, "You know what Mom? If you end up in a wheelchair like Mamaw, I'll take care of you,"

My heart sank. My daughter spoke up and said, "I will too. You'll have to move to Vegas, but I'll take care of you."

Then, at the store, without any prompting, my son picked out a sweet Thank You card that he wanted to get for my Mom. He signed his name to it when we got home and gave it to her.

My heart is full.

CHAPTER 68:
Two Pink Lines, Panic Again

June 23rd, 2022

It took 2 and a half years. I worked in 2020 in the nursing homes, and from 2021 till now, I've worked in our hospital during two surges. Not once did I contact COVID. Until now.

I tested positive yesterday (Wednesday). I had sinus issues Monday, but not terrible. I even tested myself and my son who had a nasty nose and both were negative. I'd actually just gotten over a sinus infection a week prior. Then, Tuesday evening I started to feel bad, and by yesterday morning I felt like I'd been hit by a truck. I took a test, and it was positive right away. I then tested my son, and he too is positive.

Thankfully, my husband and daughter are negative at this point. And by the grace of God, so is my mother.

I have a caregiver during the day from 8:30-5, so the exposure to her from me is at a minimum. But it's still me in the evenings and through the night (and coming weekend). I want to make sure it's still as limited as possible but protected when I do care with her. Thank God for these girls that help with my Mom. I'd be completely lost without them.

My own little daughter is amazing. I was feeling very sick yesterday, and when a friend ordered us pizza, my daughter stepped in to feed my mother so I wouldn't have to.

My son isn't terribly sick, thankfully. He just has congestion and a cough. He's not fully understanding that he can't be around anyone. Quarantining him in his room is impossible. He's outside a lot, and I have to keep an eye on him as best I can. So, no rest for me, as much as I'd like. But that's life! He's just a very active little boy, and it's killing him to see his friends outside playing, knowing he has to stay away for a week! However, he has energy and will get in the mood to clean, so I mean that's a win-win, right?

When I'm with Mom, I make sure she is protected. I wear an N95 that was graciously gifted to me, as well as gloves and eyewear. That makes taking care of her oh-so-hot! On top of that, I'm still congested and feverish, and adding that makes me almost feel sick. It's doable and we do what we have to. She still needs her teeth brushed, meds, and me taking her to/from the bathroom and putting her to bed in the evening and turning her throughout the night. That's not something that can wait or not be done. She doesn't have any symptoms, and I tested her today just to see. So far, so good for her! But we will keep watch.

I don't miss the face pain of N95's nor the shower of sweat it helps produce, but I'm thankful to keep her as protected as I can.

I'd love to just lay in bed and not be needed for a few days, but that's just not in the cards with my kids having to be at home—but apart—two dogs that are driving me crazy, and a Mom that constantly needs me.

This, too, shall pass. I already feel so much better than I had. At one point my symptoms were so severe that I should have gone to the hospital. I couldn't do that though. No one would be here to take care of Mom. I suffered through and the 104 fever and chills finally broke.

I'm lucky to be able to work from home while I'm banished from the hospital for another week - but that's frustrating because I'm used to being there. Doing what I do from home isn't fun, but I'm blessed to have the option as many don't.

I am also incredibly honored to have the kind of friends and community that I do—offering to do anything that's needed, bringing food, offering to take me to the hospital when I was sick, or just checking in constantly.

As often as I feel alone in many ways, I know I'm not.

That warms my heart—more than my fever was warming my body.

Chapter 69:
Nightmares Become Reality

June 29th, 2022

When I woke up sick and tested positive for COVID last Wednesday morning, I took action. I refused to be around my mother without an N95 mask and sanitizing. Caregivers were here during the daytime, thankfully, because my symptoms were severe.

It was the sickest I can ever remember being. So close to going to the hospital. But my husband was at work, my son was sick, as he was positive too, and my daughter locked herself in her room to stay healthy. And of course, there was Mom. But with the grace of caregivers coming to put Mom to bed for me that night, I awoke Thursday still sick, but functional.

On Friday, the congestion, cough, and fatigue were intense, but the fever and body aches were gone. Then, Mom developed her first symptom. I gave her a test, and she was positive.

My.
Heart.
Sank.

My husband also had a headache, and his home test showed a faint positive. But after two PCR tests and no worsening symptoms, it's been ruled he never did get COVID.

With Mom now positive, I wouldn't allow caregivers to come to the house. They need to protect themselves and their families at home. I couldn't do it to them. I know it's been so hard for them to be away from her. I've kept them updated just as I have our own family, because they are family.

Mom quickly deteriorated through the first evening. She began to have horrible headaches, stomach issues, and by the time I got her to bed, she was congested and running a fever.

No longer did I feel my sickness. I couldn't. I listened to her all night through the monitor and barely slept (I'm also on steroids for my COVID, so sleeping isn't a thing for me anymore). She awoke Saturday morning with fever and worsening congestion. I got out her cough assist machine—thankfully, we had that—and used it throughout the day. It did help.

Saturday I reached out to our local health officials, her doctors, and our hospital (where I work) and was able to obtain COVID antiviral pills, antibiotics, and steroids for her to begin immediately. They offered the infusion, but she refused, saying, "I'm not taking something from others with a better life ahead of them." And that was that.

By Saturday evening she was a little better, but I stayed up and wrote out preparations. I decided it was time (either because of this or the impending reality we live in) to write out first and secondary contacts for when she passes. I wrote out organizations for insurance, rentals, meds, etc. to notify upon her death. I got out her DNR and POST form, along with my POA/GUARDIAN papers and had them at the ready.

It's not dumb.
It's not morbid.
It's reality.

I know when the time comes, sooner or later, I will need all the assistance I can gather from myself now. For then. This is something I encourage everyone to do, rather you have a terminally ill loved one or not. It will make decision making less stressful on you during your time of grieving.

Come Sunday she was better. Fever was gone, congestion was lifting, and by Monday we no longer needed the cough assist. My symptoms are slightly present with sinus pressure, weakness, and fatigue (which I felt today was finally lifting), and I lost my sense of taste, which is so bizarre.

My son had a bout of coughing that led to breathing treatments. He was also placed on antibiotics and steroids due to an ongoing ear condition out of precaution, but he never got more than a snotty nose and congestion. Well, aside from a serious case of cabin fever that ultimately ended with him cutting his own hair, so we had to buzz it all off.

Quarantine is fun…

My husband and daughter remained healthy and negative. My son and I have one more day of quarantine left. Mom's tenth day is this coming Sunday, just before the 4th of July. Caregivers are coming back July 5th, which is when I physically return to work, and both kids can return to summer camp (hallelujah)!

Throughout this time, we have had so many wonderful people dropping off groceries and sending snacks, cleaning supplies, masks, and treats for the kids. I love our community and I love our village. I truly couldn't do it without them.

During this time, we also celebrated our daughter's 11th birthday. It was a COVID birthday with presents wrapped in Christmas paper (it's all we had!). I always take the kids' birthdays off work and spend the whole day doing things with just them. Because of COVID we had to postpone her birthday party, her baptism, and her birthday day off, along with not one but *three* dental appointments I'd made for the kids and Mom. So even coming out of quarantine, I'll be juggling to catch up on all of that. Not to mention, our son's 7th birthday is next week, and next weekend is now the combined birthday parties for both of the kids.

Although Mom has initially survived COVID at this point I am fearful it has weakened her and is causing her ALS to progress. Before COVID hit this past month, I'd noticed how her breathing has changed. Now, after fighting this, I can't help but think how it's drastically affected it even more so.

Yesterday and today, although no longer "sick", Mom has had a horrendous headache. She can't get rid of it. Alternating between OTC and prescription medications is not touching it. I know what that is—that's lack of oxygen.

I read a case study, and there have only been two individuals with ALS studied since the beginning of COVID. Both progressed immensely. One was even minimal in his ALS progression, had mild/moderate COVID, and within a month was late-stage ALS.

COVID may not be the end for Mom, but I'm certain it's going to play a major part.

But we keep on. I'm trying to be better in so many aspects, but when I focus on one, others suffer. I may be great at routines and organization, but I feel I lack balance. I fear my husband feels this, and our kids. When I try to focus more on that, I fear my Mom feels out of balance. It's a never ending cycle but a manageable one.

There are so many others going through such tough times that I couldn't even fathom the pain, agony, and worry they have. One in particular is my best friend. The mountains she is having to climb, that too many I know are also climbing, are overwhelming. I am the one in awe of them.

I am also in awe of my Momma. Who wouldn't be?

CHAPTER 70:
My Mindset Is Still on Full Alert

July 2nd, 2022

The changes Mom has had in the last couple of days have been very noticeable for me, so I can only imagine when someone comes (caregivers) and sees her for the first time in almost two weeks, what they're going to think.

Her terrible headache is still coming and going with little to no relief. She has taken so many OTC and prescription meds, I worry about it, but that's what she's requesting. She's very tired. More so than ever. She's very weak sounding with her voice hoarse and labored, and she just looks weak. Her eyes are weak and slightly discolored. Her weight loss is more apparent than ever. She's still eating some breakfast, lunch or a snack, and a few bites of dinner. Her intake is low, and swallowing isn't any worse, but the issue is the amount of energy it takes for her to eat. I've made cakes and got her ice cream. I'm making what I can that's easy to chew but sweet like she likes.

She says she can feel the congestion still in her chest, and you can hear it. I think it's consolidating, and the ALS is no longer allowing her to expel it even with the cough assist.

I've also noticed she's lost control of her bladder. Not so much that she's incontinent and pees while awake or asleep, but when I'm lifting her in the Hoyer, she doesn't have the muscle control to hold it until we get to the bedside toilet. So, we've had to reconfigure so I can stop doing laundry and mopping so much.

She's a little more confused and disoriented now as well. She's just so tired. This morning when I was getting her ready, she stated it didn't even feel like morning. She doesn't remember going to bed for the night. She thought I was just getting her up from a nap. "I just feel off," she told me.

I am fully aware of what the progression of the ALS she was already experiencing, and now the aftermath of COVID, has done. It's *detrimental*.

Today is her last day in quarantine; however, I don't believe the virus is there anymore. It's not like she wants to go anywhere, and there's really no one to come and see her, and that's okay. It's been nearly 2 weeks. With the holiday weekend, I'm going to try my best to make sure the kids have a good time, but focusing on her more than ever takes away from that at times.

We all return back to "normal" Tuesday with me and my husband back to work, the kids back to summer camp, and the caregivers back in the home. It's a welcome change. I could use some socialization and a breather.

I just don't think we have a "normal" to return to anymore.

CHAPTER 71:
One Year Has Passed

July 6th, 2022

One year ago today, Mom moved into our home.

I remember the day vividly. My stomach was in knots as we drove the hour north. When we got there, the movers were already there packing her things in the truck. I walked in the front doors, and there she sat in her wheelchair. Broken.

She was angry and rightfully so. As we gathered everything into the moving truck and our vehicles, Mom sat and watched. She watched as the life she had built, one she had worked so hard for and overcame so many obstacles, was being taken from her. As I loaded her into her van, she gave that gorgeous home one last look, and we pulled away. We didn't get but a mile down the road before she started to break down in sobs stating, "My life sucks, it just sucks."

She didn't mean to hurt me. *She* was hurting. The knot in my stomach tightened as we traveled on. It was a quiet ride as she cried softly, lifting the tissue up to wipe her eyes here and there. Once we reached my house, it was busy for quite a long time. The movers were moving her furniture in and placing all her boxes of belongings in our garage. *So many things*. It would take weeks for us to go through everything. To this very day, a year later, half of her things are still packed, although now in storage.

The next week was incredibly difficult. Incredibly. We had to get a routine down, and I had to learn how to use the Hoyer lift to transfer her. I remember the feeling of panic. I remember thinking I can't do this. This was a mistake. There's no way this is going to work. I had called a friend who was actually going to be a caregiver for my mom to come show me how to do things. This friend came to put my mom to bed and get her up every day for a few days until finally, I got it.

It was so hot last July (just like *this* July). It took me an hour every night to get her to bed and just as long in the mornings. I was drenched in sweat at all times. Mom was also working at that time still, so she had to be up early to get everything situated. I remember how frustrated she was that it just wasn't her space, her routine. The quiet was also gone. She had moved in with me, who at that time had two small children.

The day she moved in with us, I thought she had declined. She still had her arms, though, and her hands. The arms were starting to go, and she wasn't able to lift them very high, but she could lift them. She was still feeding herself, though it was becoming increasingly difficult. She was still typing on her laptop, holding her phone, scrolling Facebook, using the remote to change the TV channel, and using her wheelchair to move about as she pleased.

In the year that she has now lived with us, all of that is gone. Everything from the neck down is gone. She's hardly able to turn her neck. Now, after COVID, she's declined even more. She looks her age, which is something she's never done before. She's tired. Physically, emotionally, and mentally. I don't see myself doing an update this time next year titled, "Year Two of This Journey". That's just the reality.

I can look back on how things were a year ago today and be so proud of her, myself, and those around us. We have a routine down pat, and although we have to constantly make changes, they come easily to us. Her anger and frustration are now dampened by exhaustion and depression. She no longer yells at me or gets too frustrated with herself or with me. There's a type of "quiet," and although she has 24/7 care, now there's a difference with it.

This past year has been the hardest of not only her life, but mine as well. My family has put so much on hold or simply missed out because it wasn't feasible for me to leave. My children have had to share me more than they'd like, and my husband has lost a piece of me in this time as well. I'm a creature of habit and try my damndest to be as much as I can be for those I love, but there is only so much I can do at one time. That is something I still struggle with to this day.

I don't regret having Mom move in with us. It's the opposite actually. I am so very grateful that I was given the determination, the strength, and the opportunity to care for her during the last phase of her journey. She would have done the exact same thing for me in a heartbeat. Although this time has been hard on my children and they have missed out on vacations and time together with me, I hope they will look back and remember that I cared for their grandmother the way that I hoped they'd care for me. I'm praying they take away compassion, strength, determination, and drive from this experience—to give love, respect, and dignity to those we love and can help.

Their grandmother is being taken away from them. The resentment I have for ALS is real and it's rough. My mother did not get to enjoy her "golden years" the way she should have. She didn't get to travel and have new experiences. I didn't get to go shopping with her for orthopedic shoes. My kids didn't get to have sleepovers at Grandma Davis's or weekend adventures together. My mother won't be able to see them graduate high school, get married, or see how unique and terrific they will become as adults.

My kids are extremely blessed with my husband's mother—the one grandparent who is able to buy things for them, take them to the park, and have popcorn parties. The one that will be there (God willing) to watch them graduate, get married, and maybe one day hold a great-grandchild. I know many have grandparents who never got that. Heck, I'm one of them. But it's my selfish anguish that this was taken from my mother. From me.

What I don't have, however, are regrets. When my mother is gone from this Earth, I will not have one ounce of regret. Because I did everything in my power, heart, and mind to make sure she was comfortable and loved. I sacrificed just a short stint in my life to give all I could to her. My mother is truly my best friend, my confidant, and the one person in this entire world that I have looked up to so much, respected, and admired. I have her so rightfully high on a pedestal—even now as she continues to push through this phase of her life—that thinking for one moment I had ever made a mistake in putting her there is laughable.

I love her with every ounce of my being. She is very tired at this moment. I want her to be able to wake up and just be comfortable, clear-minded, and happy. We are past that. I don't see her ever coming out of this fog that she is in due to her rising CO_2. It may sound awful, but I don't want her this way. I don't want her to linger like this in a life that she never would have wanted - especially now.

My beautiful, vivacious, spunky mother is broken. I pray every day that she finds her peace.

It's been one *hell* of a year.

Temporary strife for a lifetime of gratitude, remember?

CHAPTER 72:
Caregiving for a Loved One Is Not for the Weak

July 10th, 2022

The description of my writing is, "the good, the bad, and the really ugly." I want this to show the reality of this, not only to myself as I look back, but to those of you who are reading.

Caregiving for a loved one is *not* for the weak.

That's putting it lightly. I share the hardships and the triumphs, but I'm sharing the darkness, despair, and frustration as well. Because that is the reality. It's not always rainbows and sunshine—in fact, it rarely ever is.

I get exhausted. Physically, mentally, and emotionally. More so emotionally and mentally. Having Mom 24/7 at home during this part of her journey is very time demanding.

Very.
Demanding.

No longer can I sleep in on the weekends, go where I want to go, or do what I want to do, not even around the house.

Now, before I really get into this, I'm putting in a disclaimer. I love caring for my mother. I would do this all over again without a second thought to it. But I am human. I have feelings. I express these feelings in writing as a way to vent. Not just to remember, but to share with others who are caregiving that the dark side of this is normal. Absolutely 100% normal. Feeling the frustrations and anger does *not make* you a terrible person. Yes, those we take care of cannot help that they are in full care, but we also have a right to feel what we feel when we do it.

When I am home with Mom, my name is called a hundred times during a 24-hour period. Throughout the day and throughout the night. Whether I am cooking, cleaning, or sitting to read a book or watch a show, I legit cannot finish a task without my name being called for help.

Help consists of wiping her eyes that are running, swiping hair from her face, flossing her teeth because something is stuck, picking her nose because she has boogers, adjusting her bottom because it's hurting, or her elbow, or her feet, or her hands.

I am my mother's physical body.

I will be boiling water and my name is called. I'll be watching something my kids want to show me, and my name is called. If she doesn't know where I am or hear from me (God forbid I sit down and read) then she's calling for me. This has made me get into the habit of telling her my every move. If I'm going to the bathroom, I tell her. If I'm going to start laundry, dinner, or clean something, I tell her. That has become more of a catch-22 because I'll mention to her, "I'm going to the bathroom," but she'll stop me from doing something right then. Sometimes that something is quick, but other times it's not and I'm about to pee my pants before it's said and done.

The other night I was watching a movie with my daughter while Mom was in bed, and we had to pause the movie *six times* because I was called into her room. If she hears a noise, she calls me to ask what it is. If she doesn't hear the dogs, she makes me stop what I am doing to go check on them. This also goes if she doesn't hear the kids. If I make a loud noise (getting pans out) she's calling out to ask what's happening. If the dogs are barking, she's having me stop and see what they're barking at. That's added to her calling me over to adjust something or tend to her needs.

That's what a caregiver does. However, it's 24/7, and I get irritated and frustrated. Today my husband is napping on the couch. I *loathe* him. I wanted to do just that. I did a little experiment and have counted how many times I got up to tend to her just from 2:00pm to 3:30pm. The number was twenty-eight. *Twenty-eight*. In just a little over an hour.

I can leave Mom for about an hour at a time sometimes, as long as she doesn't have to use the restroom. That's allowed me— *allowed me*—to attend church and run to the grocery sometimes.

Thank goodness for grocery pick-up. My family hasn't been out to eat since she moved in. I can't just go shopping for kids' clothes or browse around. I typically don't leave my house from Friday when I get home from work until Monday when I go to work.

Oh, thank God I work. I'd never be able to do this if I didn't get to leave five days a week for about eight hours and be at work. Thank *God* for the caregivers that come in. Work is my sanity. When we were home for two weeks with COVID, I didn't think we were going to mentally make it, and by "we," I mean "me."

Now.

Now that I've vented the all-consuming frustration, I do want to again note that my mother cannot help it. She did not ask for ALS. She hates this. *Hates it.* I do my best not to ever show my frustration, and I'm pretty good at it. Even when she snaps, when she asks me to do something and I reply, "I'll be there in a second, just need to finish this," her getting angry and saying, "You know, I can't help it," isn't her actually being angry at *me*. It's her anger towards ALS. And I know that.

I would take care of her all over again in a heartbeat. I just wanted to share that feelings of despair, anger, and frustration are completely normal and will happen.

I usually put that in perspective. I take a deep breath and do whatever it is she needs me to do. Because, once again, this isn't going to be forever.

CHAPTER 73:
Trapped in Her Own Body

July 30th, 2022

Mom has been sleeping *so* much this last week. I got her up for about 30 minutes today, and she needed to go right back to bed. She's awfully tired and hurts all over, especially headaches and back pain. Her neck is now contracting more to one side, and she can't lift her head very well because it hurts. At this point she can move her mouth, nose, and eyes with sometimes a little nudge of her head. That's it.

It's getting harder to swallow, so she's barely eating. From the beginning, she has refused the feeding tube and trach. She's a 73-year-old retired nurse. She knows.

Can you imagine?

Without ever experiencing it, I'm guessing you can't. *I* can't and I see it every day. The thoughts of how being trapped within your own body keep me awake sometimes. The fear, the hurt, the frustration that must coil inside oneself. My mother is the strongest person I have ever met, hands down. She has taken this death sentence with grace, with grit, and with an outlook that no average human ever could. I know I couldn't.

I just can't help but to feel that we are on the down-slide, you know? I've talked about it before, but I just have this feeling inside of me I can't explain. It's not panic or even grief. It's calm. A peace.

Upon her request, yesterday she had someone come and perform the Anointing of the Sick for her. It used to be called the "last rites," but it's changed to where it's not necessarily for someone on their deathbed, but rather to be performed while the person is sick and conscious. Sometimes praying for healing of what ails them, but also for those seeking healing of their soul. This was what Mom wanted.

I'm thankful I was able to arrange that for her. All I can aspire to do is provide whatever she needs or wants during this part of her ALS journey.

Chapter 74:
Choking Up

August 22, 2022

Mom has been choking much more often lately. We've noticed it more in the evenings, which my common sense tells me is because the muscles in her throat are weaker at the end of the day.

She chokes every night at supper. No matter how fine the meat or how sauced anything is. We made cereal the other night, and she aspirated some. Tonight, it was oatmeal.

Tonight was worse than ever, though, because she just couldn't swallow without choking, even as I was getting her ready for bed. Choking in her chair, in the Hoyer, on the toilet, and in the bed. *Two hours* of this.

Yesterday she was so tired that she went to bed at four in the afternoon. She didn't call me once. Before I went to bed, I turned her, and she didn't even wake up. Throughout the night, I noticed her breathing was weirder than usual. Shallower, more gasp-like at times. I turned her again when I got up at 2am with my son, who had a nightmare, and then again before I left for work. She doesn't remember it at all.

She was a little more alert today, so I thought we'd have a better evening. Yet, at dinner time there was a lot of choking again.

We are probably going to start to take her multitude of nightly pills with pudding instead of the water. She choked like crazy on her meds tonight. Even utilizing the techniques for swallowing deterioration (pudding, crushing meds, etc.), I don't think it's going to help.

She's still losing weight, not only because of the choking, but because she just doesn't have an appetite. Nothing sounds good. *Nothing.* I hate that more than anything really.

I'm still scrambling here and there with her appointments, caregiver schedules, my work, the kids appointments, and their ongoing extracurricular activities. I'm really just on autopilot at this point. I've taken up reading again, and I'm flying through books, only having the time to read once everyone else is in bed. Then I'm up past midnight because my brain is soaking in the stories and relaxation that comes with a good book.

Escaping my stress. That's what reading is doing for me at this point. I write to express my stress and then I read other's works to escape it.

CHAPTER 75:
Emotional Punching Bag

August 25, 2022

Even when the crap is hitting the fan as her body continues to fail her, we somehow still find a way. I can't do anything about her choking more frequently than not (she choked twice this evening), but I did find a solution for when we are taking her down the ramp. Since she doesn't have control of her neck muscles, when going down the ramp in her chair her neck would snap forward and hang, which hurt her, of course.

I used one of my stretchy headbands that went around her headrest and her forehead! Now when she goes down, her neck doesn't thrust forward. It was so hard last night that she cried. That was it. I had to do something. I went to our ALS Facebook forum for advice, and someone suggested this method and it worked.

I still have a few other options, but for now this method is working for us.

Mom had a dental cleaning today. I'm not sure when it happened, but sometime between the time when she got up and when we left for the dentist, she became severely agitated. *Everything* was pissing her off. I could tell it in her eyes, her expressions, and her tone.

Quite frankly, she bit my head off more times today than she has in months. She didn't want to wear the neck brace on the way to the dentist (the one that goes under her chin) because she didn't think it would help. But then on the way to the appointment I had to drive with one hand and hold her head back with the other. Reclining the chair back a little did help; however, I hit the button too long and it hit her feet.

I know it hurt, but she ripped into me like I'd done it on purpose. Then at the doctor, she wanted her chair to tilt back while we waited, which was no problem. But when they called her, I had to put it down some, because if it's back at a certain point it won't roll forward, and she was yelling at me to go back more. I tried to explain I couldn't, and she just got even more upset.

Then this evening, she needed to use the restroom, so I was trying to hurry, but there's a lot that goes into undressing her and getting her on the Hoyer. When I got her up into it and over to the bedside toilet, she began to yell at me again to hurry and put her down, but I can go only as fast as the Hoyer will allow.

When she has to be moved over or adjusted, she hurts. I get it. Tonight though, as I was doing the usual adjusting things, she cried out in anger and said I didn't have to be so rough. Telling me I can't push her using her shoulders, arms, neck, back, or ribs.

So, unless I can manifest the ability of telekinesis, I'm not sure what I can do here.

Through all of that, I didn't say anything. I didn't bark back. Because I do understand she is not angry at *me*. She's angry at ALS. She's angry at her failing body. She has *every* right to cuss, scream, throw a fit, or whatever. It's well warranted. I know this.

I am also human. I honestly do feel her frustrations. I get frustrated too. We are both making incredible sacrifices, and we are both fueled by the emotions of this journey.

I'm telling anyone out there who is taking care of a loved one who's hurt or ill—we are *allowed* to also feel the grief, the anger, the agitation, and the frustration. We are human, and if you're caring for someone else, then you're already invested in all the good, the bad, and more so the ugly that goes along with their journey.

It's our journey too.

CHAPTER 76:
It's Been a Lot Lately

August 9th, 2022

A. LOT.

Mom's swallowing issues and choking has increased to the point that she is no longer able to swallow her medicine, especially in the evening. We have had two instances where oxygen was lost, and she aspirated.

So, I was able to obtain a pestle and mortar to crush her medicine. She hates the taste with it in applesauce (pudding didn't work well) but at least she isn't choking on them anymore.

On top of that issue, food as well has become worse. She's barely eating because either she chokes, or she's completely lost her appetite. That one kills me. Not even the flavor or enjoyment of a meal or snack does she have to look forward to anymore. Just one more way her body continues to fail her.

On top of *that*, her head control is terrible. She has what they call "head drop" so badly that it's painful for her. We have utilized the support strap for when she's in her chair, especially going down the ramp. Now we are faced with the issue when it comes to using the bedside toilet.

Her head hangs so low, not only is it painful, her nose then completely runs. Then she chokes on the drainage. So tonight, she's using the restroom, her head is hanging down and she starts to choke on the drainage, as she's using the restroom. For thirty minutes I stood next to the bedside toilet and held her head back. We have a collar that is supposed to help but it doesn't work well, and she can't take how uncomfortable it is.

Frustrating. That's what it is.

I'm frustrated that this keeps piling on her and we are running out of ideas and tricks to fix it as it happens. Without the feeding tube we are at the last of what we can do medicine and food wise. She is in constant need of assistance. I'm glad to give it and anything I can to her.

More to her means less for my family and myself. That sounds and feels terrible to even write, but once again I'm human. I want to be able to do so much but I am limited because of my responsibilities. Yes, I chose this, and I would again and again; however, I'm exhausted.

This week has been a lot on the home front. It'll even out again, but until we can figure out a normal with these changes, I'm just buckling up and holding on for the ride.

I've said it more than once and I'll keep saying it—fuck ALS.

Chapter 77:
A Harsh Reality

September 19th, 2022

"If I could, I would just roll myself off a cliff."

Tensions are mounting. I guess I shouldn't say tensions—more like frustrations and tensions. From both mom and myself. I have to wonder, as much as I try to keep myself from showing my frustrations or tensions in front of her, if perhaps she's absorbing what I'm silently fighting inside.

I hate being home. I hate coming home from work. I hate being home from Friday after work until I leave again on Monday. I no longer look forward to weekends because it's not a break. I work mentally and physically harder at home than I do in my career. My job? It's my "me time." It's my break.

That's the harsh reality, and my writing I had promised—would be the good, the bad and the really ugly. Right now, it's really ugly. *Super ugly.*

I shouldn't have to preface this, but I will. I am sympathetic to my mother's disease. My ranting and ravings are how I, as a human, deal with human emotions that come along with being the caregiver for my ALS mother. Although I may vent and scream, I am eternally grateful to be able to care for her during this tortuous journey. The thing is—this journey is not just hers alone. It belongs to me, my family, and everyone else involved.

Mom has never been a "please" and "thank you" person. Although she is compassionate and loving, she's just never been very outwardly affectionate, not to the degree my father was or the degree to which I am. Don't get me wrong, when I was sick or hurt, she was *very* comforting. Mom has a temper. Mom doesn't have much patience. Add in this terrible disease, and that's amped by a thousand.

When I am home, evenings, nights, and all weekend long, it's Mom commanding me to do something. Constantly. Move this, do this, fix this, over and over. When I tell you I do not sit down for more than a five minute time span, I'm not lying. She is *obsessed* with our two puppies.

Do they have water?
Do they have food?
What are they chewing on?
Why are they barking?
Why are they quiet?
Where are they?

She cannot help it, I know. Again, I am sympathetic. However, this frustration that I cannot do anything I'm wanting or needing to do, whether it's chores, something with the kids or my husband, just sit and read a book, or go anywhere whenever I want, well it mounts up.

This happens occasionally. Not as often as one would think. Unlike my mom, I do have patience. But also, like my mom, I am a person. It gets to the point where I am so tense on the inside I could just scream. Sometimes I do.

Sometimes I find myself sitting in my van in the driveway and just screaming at the top of my lungs. It's a release. It helps. As the mounting tension comes, it is soon released, and I'm good for another month or so before it piles on again.

I feel guilty when I am this way. I am snapping at my kids, my husband, and anyone else around me. I hate it. It's naive to think she doesn't see this, even though I work hard not to make a face and I watch my tone. Mom knows me.

She didn't want this for me either - but we are here, together.

"This is no life," she told me today. Tomorrow is her ALS clinic, and she usually gets emotional during this time. She doesn't want to live this way, her body constantly failing her, but it just will not let her go.

I never, in a million years, thought I'd be praying for my mother to not wake up.

Until you yourself have gone through a terminal disease like ALS, or until you are the caregiver for someone with that disease, it's very hard to truly comprehend. Wishing for death is not cruel, and it doesn't mean you won't miss the person. Wishing for death is not cruel. It does not mean you will not miss the person.

There comes a time where quality is worth far more than quantity, but there is also a time where the quality ends no matter how hard you try. I feel as if we are there within our journey. Can she progress more without passing away?

Yes.

She can lose her ability to speak as her voice is already weak. She can start salivating and drooling on herself. She can lose the ability to close or open her eyes and mouth. There are still plenty of ways her body can fail her, even though she's already paralyzed from the neck down and unable to move her head or hold it up. She chokes constantly on her food and on pills that we cannot crush. Yet, there is still room for *more* torture.

I won't get started again on the Right to Die/Death with Dignity. Not now. Everything I have said is the 100% reason why all 50 states should pass it though.

I am not alone on this journey in the compass of support. We have wonderful caregivers Monday thru Friday from 8am until 5pm. Because of them, I can work. Because of them, I get that break. As we approach 15 months since she moved in with us, Mom has now begun to save a lot of her discomforts for when the caregiver leaves. She says she doesn't want to bother them if she can wait until I walk through the door.

I get home from work with the kids, trying to juggle the insane doodles, get dinner started for everyone, and yet I'm called constantly to her. I'm usually good at managing, but at this moment I am not. It'll go away, and we will find the balance yet again.

It's always there waiting for me to rediscover it—the balance.

Just writing this out helps so much. Sharing it publicly, not for sympathy or even bragging rights (how in the hell does this get confused as *bragging*), but sharing it to show other caregivers that we are human, our feelings are valid, and we shouldn't feel guilty (we will) or ashamed (we will) when the tension mounts up.

Also, I don't share this with my mother. She doesn't need to know my inner demons or my struggles. She has her own.

That's been truly the hardest thing. My mother has always been my rock, the person I turn to, vent to, discuss everything with. This, I cannot share with her. I won't. Which means I don't have the one person I need to talk this through with.

She's calling me again. I've started and stopped writing this chapter six times in a forty-five minute time-span because I've had to go to her. Yet, because I got it out here in the writing world, the smile I'll have on my face when I come to her won't actually be forced.

Chapter 78:
Decisions Have Been Made

September 22nd, 2022

Hospice.

For many, that is such a scary word. We resonate that word with dying. It's so much more though.

Mom had her quarterly ALS Clinic a few days ago and was confronted by her ALS team with the recommendation for hospice. Due to her continued decline and the end stage of her disease, it is time. Mom wasn't expecting to hear that from them. Although we had discussed it together, hearing it from her physicians really put things into perspective for her.

I watched her after that clinic. I watched her the following days. I saw the internal struggle through her eyes, the wrestling of her emotions, and the realization of her reality. It was torturous for me. I felt she looked defeated, but I believe what I saw was her final acceptance.

Today, she agreed to be put on hospice services here at home.

Many patients can live on hospice for quite some time. Others find that, once they accept it, their body does too, and they are freed.

Freed.

When my mother passes, an unmendable hole will be created in my life and inside my heart. But as much grief and pain as I know is coming for me, I know it will be a release for her. She will not have lost her battle with ALS, no. Her passing will be her victory of this disease.

Given our career paths of nursing home administration, we both are well-versed in hospice. We have both had the conversation with family members of our residents about hospice many times. Somehow, being on this end of it is very different.

I can't say sadness has come over me since her decision. It's been more like shock at yet another step, another transition. *The* transition. Nothing has changed from yesterday to today, and yet everything now feels different. Putting her to bed tonight, our conversation and tone with reality was noticeable.

We have always been preparers. Always.

She'd mentioned earlier this evening that I need to make sure I have a list of places to contact once she's passed, like social security, the army, insurances, and so on. "Mom, I did that this summer when you had COVID."

She said to make sure I have a list of people, family and friends, to contact. "Done already."

When I was putting her to bed she said to me, "You know, you don't even know what I want to be buried in." She laughed when I replied, "A cardboard box, right?" But then I looked at her and said, "One of your nice dress suits you always wore to work." She smiled.

She forgot we'd had this conversation when my dad passed away. I have a list of everything down to her flowers and her music. We are preparers.

I also realize *nothing* will prepare me for losing my mother. It's a trauma I haven't gone through, so I can't be prepared. We've been grieving since her diagnosis, yes, but facing the reality that she will leave this earth sooner rather than later, well, I don't think you can prepare for it. You can only feel it in real-time.

We will still laugh every day. I will make sure she gets to enjoy what foods sound even half-way good and let her tolerate it as best she can. Which means a whole lot of ribeyes, baked potatoes, fried potatoes, sweet butter corn, ham and beans, potato soup, banana pudding, and banana splits.

I have done everything in my power to care for her, and nothing will change that. We have our wonderful caregivers, and now we can open our hearts to a few more on that list with the hospice aide and hospice nurse that will be beside us, along with our girls, the rest of the way *home*.

Chapter 79:
I Had to Leave Work

October 12, 2022

Mom choked and aspirated today.

She's been choking for months, increasingly so every day that has passed. We'd gotten to the point that we crushed her meds and didn't get so alarmed when she'd have a spasm of "coughing" while eating—no matter what it was, how thin, or how thick. I say "coughing" because ALS has long deteriorated her diaphragm, so her cough is barely there.

I got a call at work from our caregiver when Mom's coughing fit didn't stop this morning. I came home, and she was still having trouble. I contacted the hospice nurse, and she came right away. She could tell there wasn't much air movement in her lower left lung, and she suggested we go to the hospital to get a chest X-ray done just to see what we are working with and then talk about decisions.

On the way to the hospital, Mom was actually able to cough up something, so we think it was dislodged because her X-ray in the ER was clear of any foreign items. We feel that the damage was done though. Mom was okay for a bit but then started into a fit again, unable to move much air and coughing so much. Her heart rate would go high and her O2 low, and it stayed that way for a bit.

They gave her a shot of Valium, and that eventually seemed to help, as she's resting now and the coughing has stopped. It's a very good possibility that she'll continue to cough, since she already has a buildup of mucus too far down for the suction to reach. We have a patch behind her ear to hopefully help dry it up some.

We're told this is quite possibly the beginning of the end. If she can't go back to how she was, if today is her new normal, well then, I pray it is quick. It's terrible to see the woman you love and admire more than anyone on this earth struggle to catch her breath.

We have our hospice team and our meds ready to go because I'll be damned if she suffers. We knew this was where our journey was leading us. We are arriving at our final destination. Maybe not today, maybe not tomorrow, but I feel it in my heart that we've taken the last exit and are approaching the end.

This rests well within my soul. We've grieved for so long. We've faced the reality of her mortality from the moment of diagnosis. It isn't fair, but what aspect of life is? I have learned so much, grown so much, and evolved more than I ever thought possible during this journey with her.

I will *never* regret this time. I will mourn all the things we never got to do or that she'll never get to see, but I will never mourn *this*. Being next to her, right by her side, the whole way.

She's better this evening. The coughing has stopped. She was able to eat some oatmeal and take her meds. I've already had to give her some extra pain meds.

I just wish there was a sign that was definitive and said, "This is it." I feel like a yo-yo lately. Is this it? Is it not? Nope, we are good? Wait, no we aren't? When it comes to notifying friends and family, I'm starting to feel like the Boy Who Cried Wolf, but I'd rather raise a false alarm a few times than be silent at what might be the crucial moment.

Catch-22, right there.

CHAPTER 80

Hypervigilant in My Observations

October 14, 2022

Things progressed and changed yesterday. Wednesday after she aspirated and I got her to bed, it was a pretty normal night. I had put a patch behind her ear to help with her phlegm, and she wanted some pain medicine around midnight.

When I got up yesterday, she was still asleep, and her breathing was a little different. I took her oxygen level, and it was 72. That's low. While getting her up, she was very disoriented and confused, and she could hardly stay awake to get into her chair. The hospice nurse came by, and her blood pressure was 90/42. That's low.

She wasn't making sense even when she was awake and speaking. She was hallucinating. She was asleep but talking silently to someone who wasn't there. She also was pretending she was eating.

I like to think she's on a dinner date with my dad.

As the day progressed, she became a little more alert, which I was thankful for because her sisters from Kentucky came. One of my brothers came, although the one is still in jail. Both of my sisters came as well. She went to bed, and the night was uneventful.

When she slept, she would gasp and grunt occasionally, but she seemed peaceful. Her oxygen levels were in the high 80's and low 90's. She didn't call for me at all, but I turned her a few times while she slept. I also slept on the couch in the den by her room so I'd be as close as I could be to her.

Today, she is still very confused and groggy. She's still talking nonsense. Her blood pressure was 104/56, so low but not *as* low. Her oxygen is staying in the mid 90's too, but her breaths are shallow.

She's so peaceful, though. She's so pleasant and *happy*. It's weird. She's loving seeing people, and she's just so pleasantly confused. It's a relief. She's in no pain. She's in no distress.

It's possible we are working on the dying process, but there isn't a flashing signal saying, "HERE IT IS." We know we don't have months. I feel as if we don't have weeks. All I know for certain is our time is now limited.

ALS has taken everything physically from her. The only thing left for it to take was her breath and her voice.

CHAPTER 81:
Harsh Realizations

October 15, 2022

Mom hasn't had much of a change. Her oxygen levels seem to hold steady in the low 90's. Yesterday, she remained confused for the most part, not making much sense or going from one place to another when talking. She's still very tired, so I'm trying not to keep her up in her chair as much as she wants to be. The evenings are always better for clarity for some reason, but she's still talking out of her head quite a bit.

She had some bites of a banana split in the afternoon, which is her favorite. For supper she wanted fried chicken. I grimaced because the risk of her choking is so much greater now. She could eat about five bites before it was too dangerous to go on. Then, when taking her meds (crushed in applesauce) she choked and aspirated again. First time ever she choked on that. Tonight, I plan to do as much medicine by liquid and lessen what I can get crushed.

A realization hit me yesterday when it was just me and her for about fifteen minutes (we've got a lot of family here). She was talking to me but wasn't making any sense. I listened to her, nodding my head and smiling when she would, or raising my eyebrows in surprise when she would, as if I was following right along.

The realization? I'm never going to have a normal conversation with my Momma again.

That actually brought tears to my eyes. I didn't cry, not yet, but that hurt my heart deeply.

No more advice on cooking, how to deal with kiddos and life, or work-related things. No more being told how dirty my house is, no more hearing stories of her and Dad.

I am used to ALS taking everything physically from her, but this is different. She's still in good spirits. She isn't questioning why everyone is here coming to see her, which is *not* her. She's just accepting it with a smile. She's no longer always cold and hasn't even worn much of a blanket in two days. She's not in pain or in any distress. I believe we are at a new normal here, but I'm not sure for how long.

Not sure how long someone can remain alive with such high CO_2 build up. She's technically entering respiratory failure which is how 90% of ALS patients pass. Although oxygen is decent, her breathing is shallow.

It's a transition of sorts, one I wasn't expecting. I'm so happy she's like this and not in agonizing pain or distress. I have grieved for her physical form since diagnosis. However, I already miss my mother in the aspect of mentality. This is a whole new kind of grief.

I'd give anything for her to point out the cobwebs in the corners.

CHAPTER 82:
Later the Same Day

October 15, 2022

I mentioned earlier today how I had realized I would never have another normal conversation with Momma.

Today's changes were massive. At first this morning, I couldn't wake Mom at all. She was breathing okay but wouldn't respond to my touch or my voice. I waited and tried again later, and finally got her eyes to open. Ever since she moved in, Momma was adamant that I get her up no later than 9am on the weekends. No matter what. She wasn't going to lay in bed all day. This has been hardwired into my brain.

Today she didn't want to get up. She couldn't stay awake, and when she *was* awake, she was confused and disoriented. She could recognize people, but we had no idea what she was saying. I felt off all day long with her in bed and not up in her chair. I felt like I was going to get in trouble, that she was going to get super angry at me when she realized I let her stay in bed all day. It was such an odd feeling.

Finally, around 5:00pm, the hospice nurse was here, and we tried to get Mom to use the restroom. It had been well over 24 hours, and if she couldn't go on her own, we would have to get it for her by using a straight catheter. Hearing that would be the next step did it for mom, and not only was she able to use the restroom, she got up in her chair for a while.

She sat in the den and visited with the family members who had come in to see her. Again, she was alert but not making much sense. She'd start with one story, and it'd go upside down, left, and right, and then she'd forget what she was saying or forget she was talking at all. She even made a few comments about how confused she was.

Around 7pm, she was ready to lay back down. It was just me and her as I started our process of getting her to bed. Then, something happened that took me completely off guard.

She said to me, "I heard what they were saying about me. I heard about the 3-6 months. Don't lie to me Cassie."

I looked at her, *really* looked at her and said, "Like you have 3-6 months to live?" She nodded her head yes. I took a breath and told her that there was only one person that knew when we would die. She asked who that was, and I replied, "God."

"I mean clinically, Cassie, what are they saying? Just tell me."

There she was. It was my mom. She was completely lucid. I took a breath and was honest with her. We have always been honest with each other.

I told her, "Signs are pointing that we will be lucky to have a week at most, Momma." I could see the realization roll across her expression. She asked what her vital signs were, which tonight her blood pressure was 96/54, oxygen was at 92, and pulse was somewhere in the low 70's, which wasn't so terrible.

Momma looked at me and asked, "Does everyone know?" And I said yes, Momma, that's why everyone has been here. She looked at me and said, "I choked pretty bad." Again, I agreed with a nod of my head. I continued our process of getting ready for bed when she said, "The insurance, and the policy…"

But I made her stop and said to her, "Momma, it's okay. I've got everything together just like you told me to. Everything is taken care of because you prepared for this. We have prepared for this, remember?"

Momma looked right at me and said, "You've taken such good care of me. I'm going to be able to take that with me."

My whole body just froze. My chest tightened.

Then, she was gone again. She started talking about carpets and vans.

I got that normal conversation with my Momma after all.

CHAPTER 83:
Is This Really *It?*

October 16, 2022

I've been wrestling with the question of, "Is this really it?" since she aspirated Wednesday. Thursday was the worst day. Friday wasn't great. Yesterday was terrible.

Today? Today she got up by 9am, a little confused but mostly short-term memory issues. She ate some of her breakfast without any issues. She sat and visited with the crowd of family that came by. She was lucid pretty much most of the time, more like her old self with *not* enjoying so many people talking at once. Mom never really enjoyed a full house unless it was a holiday, and that was only for about two hours tops.

The only thing today that stood out was how tired she was. She went to bed at 3:45 in the afternoon but honestly could have gone to bed by noon with the way she was looking. Blood pressure and oxygen were steady today.

I come from the world of long-term care. I know healthcare. I know that many people, when dying, have their "rally" period, when you think they're passing and then have a really good day. Sometimes it's numerous days or a week, and then just when you think you're in the clear, they're gone.

I'm just not sold that this is what today *actually* was. I'm not sold that Momma didn't rebound from the aspiration complications. No one can give a time frame. Hospice can give theirs, but really, as they said, it's up to her and God.

She has no memory of the last few days, maybe some snippets here and there. That's the CO_2, I am sure. Each night holds a sense of anticipation akin to Christmas Eve, as I never know what the next day will bring. If she's clear headed tomorrow, then I'll know she's on her way back. I think.

I sound like an impatient child. I'm wanting to know an impossible answer and wanting to know it *now*. I don't know why. I know she's had a decline, and even though she may be charging her way back up, I know she'll never regain everything.

These past few days, we've gotten prepared for it. Family has been here to see her. I've gotten pictures out of storage to put together for a funeral visitation. I got out one of her favorite work outfits to have her dressed in. I've reached out to the funeral home and life insurance to ensure everything is, in fact, in place.

That won't be for nothing. Even if it's not needed for weeks or months from now, at least it's together and confirmed. I won't have to deal with it at the time, and many in the family were able to visit with her on a "good" day for their memories.

I'm learning to just take each day by stride. Her time is limited—that is for sure. If you know my Momma, you know that if someone is saying she has a certain amount of time, then she's going to say, "watch this," and take the lead doing it on her own terms. As she should. As she has her whole life. I'm just here for the ride.

CHAPTER 84:
This Is Exhausting

October 20, 2022

I thought the last 15 months of our journey was something. I had *no idea,* compared to what these last 8 days have been. It's been 8 days since Mom aspirated and started this spiral of decline. I haven't returned to work since that day. I've been right by her side.

Since then, she's had good days and bad days, although her good days haven't been anything like they were before she choked. Good days meant she got out of bed, she wasn't talking out of her head, and was alert. She would try and eat, although every time she did, she choked and even aspirated multiple times. Bad days meant she was confused and disoriented, staying in bed and barely able to be awake. Not eating or drinking.

Today was the worst day we've had. Ever. Not only since her recent decline, but since her diagnosis altogether.

Everything with Mom is slowing down on the inside. The assistance needed today with our amazing hospice nurse to alleviate issues with the restroom went far and beyond anything Momma has ever had to do or I have had to witness. Even then, not everything was relieved, which tells us her GI motility has ceased. They can't hear any sounds in her belly or feel her muscles pushing. Although on the other end, after being catheterized, she did feel relief there. Unfortunately, even though she hadn't peed since 9:30 yesterday morning, her bladder did not have very much in it, which tells us her kidneys aren't functioning properly.

She hasn't been able to get out of bed today. The movements today to try and give her relief completely drained her. She is shorter of breath today than ever before. Her resting heart rate is in the 120's. Her body temperature is wonky, and her knees are discolored.

She hasn't eaten today and has only had a few sips of water to help alleviate her dry throat.

We placed a pain patch on her this evening to help with pain. The only other medicine she has taken is liquid pain meds. Our discussion when she moved in was that I wouldn't allow her to be in pain or gasping for air. I intend to uphold that promise to her.

Today I started to break emotionally. Not a full breakdown, but the force of what is happening to my mother was weighing on me. Not the fact that she's going to be gone, although no one can fully prepare you for that. The agony she felt today, the misery she was in—it was as though I were feeling it too. I was overwhelmed, and all the while my son was begging me to take them out to breakfast. I finally was comfortable leaving Mom around 2pm today to get out with them for a few hours. They needed it. I needed it.

I need my brother, the one who still remains in jail. My heart sinks like a rock into the pit of my stomach knowing that what she said was true when he'd been arrested earlier this year: She'd never see him again.

It breaks me *for* my brother. Knowing the emotional turmoil he's experiencing with the knowledge that his mother is dying and he's not here with her. It also angers me. Selfishly it angers me because *I* need him. I don't want to have to go through this without him, yet I have to. Addiction is terrible for the addict and for those who love them.

Thoughts of knowing the end is approaching don't concern me more than I just want her to be comfortable. Tonight, she told me she finally was, so thankfully the pain meds are starting to work for her.

I catch myself with glitches of that thought. My Momma is leaving. Working toward this part of her journey has always been a mix of emotions. I want her free of this terrible disease.

This disease has robbed her of her golden years. Robbed us of having her watch my children graduate, get married, become themselves. Robbed me of all of that as well. There is anger and despair, but I've always been taught to deal with whatever life hands me.

You must accept the things you cannot change and have the wisdom to know the difference. AA has got it on point with that one.

These are the same thoughts that always made me lose my breath when my father passed ten years ago—the fact that he no longer existed in this world. I'd never hear his voice, feel his touch, or see his face. It always sat like a rock in my stomach. That's where my mind is trying to take me now with my mother.

This is it. This is the final transition to the final fatal stage of ALS.

No amount of research, advocating, planning, or praying will ever prepare you for the reality that lies within this stage of finality.

I just pray I am able to lead her through the rest of her journey with the dedication, compassion, strength, and grace that have always made my mother who she is.

CHAPTER 85:
I'm Going to Miss Her Soon

October 22, 2022

We had a rough evening. Momma hasn't been out of bed since Wednesday, and it is now Saturday. Yesterday she did eat a little bit of soup and started taking morphine and Ativan, as she was having some pain with breathing and her heart rate was elevated.

I always thought when you give someone morphine, they're knocked out–but not Mom. She rested but was alert most of the day. She didn't feel comfortable getting her nighttime meds, she just kept with the morphine. The hospice nurse placed a Foley catheter yesterday because momma doesn't have the strength to get up anymore. Plus, when she does, it's harder to breathe and her heart races.

We noticed her output of urine is very minimal, and what output there has been is very dark brown and unbelievably foul in odor (this isn't TMI—this writing is also for educational purposes). This was explained by the nurse that her kidneys are shutting down.

Last night, the morphine doses she received would take the edge off the pain but wouldn't alleviate it. Around 4am this morning, she was hurting *really* bad. She hadn't had her medicine for nerve pain in a few days, so I crushed it up and gave it to her, then brushed her teeth to get the nasty taste out of her mouth. That seemed to help some, but she agreed for us to up her morphine dose today, as well as her pain patch. I remember when my mother couldn't even really take ibuprofen. She was never one to take much medication, especially pain medication.

We gave her a bath this morning and washed her hair. She was rubbed down with her favorite scented lotion. I brushed her teeth again, changed her pajamas and her bedding. Since then and with the increase of her morphine, she has rested so much better.

She is alert when you talk to her, although her eyes aren't always opening. Her chest no longer rises when she breathes, just her stomach. This was a sign of decline the hospice nurse had told us about.

It was during this time that she spoke to me. I told her I love her, and she repeated that she loved me too. Her voice was a little softer than usual, almost a whisper, and her eyes never opened. I leaned over to her, kissed her forehead, and told her it was okay—that I loved her and that *I was going to be okay.* She opened her eyes just a little and whispered, "I'll always be with you, honey."

Momma is making her way to my Daddy, and she will be reunited with him soon.

It's funny to me that the last ten days have been such a yo-yo with her decline. She's worse, she's better. This is it, no it's not. I'm hopeful that her suffering is coming to an end, then happy to have another chance to talk to her. And then it's back and forth all over again.

Now, though, it is truly happening. There will be very little chance for a rally at this point forward. I find myself in my clinical state of mind that it could be any minute to days. Then again, this is my Momma we are talking about.

Due to her increase in decline and decrease in awareness, I made the decision to have my brother in jail call me. It broke my heart to explain to him that this was truly happening, that our momma was leaving us. The guttural cry over the phone shattered me, and I could barely talk through my tears to him. I told my brother that I was going to put him on speakerphone, that he needed to tell her that he loved her. She *needed* to hear his voice. When my mother heard her youngest son's voice come through the phone, the smile on her face widened as she told him how much she loved him. It broke my brother. I know it did.

In retrospect, dealing with his addiction had my brother almost miss saying goodbye to our father 10 years prior after having been arrested on his way to see our dad in the hospital. Although I am 12 years younger, this brother has always been close to me. I left our dying father's bedside and rushed to bail my brother out of jail and bring him to the hospital. He was able to be beside our dad as he left this world. He was able to attend his funeral. This time, with our mother, there is no bail. There is no chance for him to be here beside her, *beside me*. I tried. I called in as many favors as I could within our local judicial system, but it wasn't a possibility in letting him out for this. Given his current situation, this phone call was the best I could do to give my brother his chance to say his goodbyes.

Mom's ALS doctor had stated she was far more progressed than any of their current patients that didn't have a feeding tube or trach. My response to that? "Momma never does anything half-assed." She rode this journey to the very end, exhausting *everything* that ALS had to take from her, and she has done so with bravery, diligence, dignity, and grace.

I'm going to miss her.

That is the *most* generic statement I could make at this point.

Today, my chest has become heavy, and that familiar pit in my stomach has begun to ball up just like it had done when I lost my dad. I've cried, even broken down a couple times. Thankfully, my husband has taken the kids out for the afternoon for some fun. I needed these first moments of tears to be in private. There will be more to come. Many. More.

That is how I know, truly in my heart, that she is leaving now. God is preparing me. I have always had faith and trusted in His journey for me. This is His way of letting me get it out so that I do not have a complete breakdown when she's called *home*. Because there will be things to do, and I have to be the one to do them.

Momma has always told me to "suck it up and deal with it." If you don't like how things are, only *you* can change that. If there is nothing you can do to change it, then you adapt. You meet the challenge as best as you can and create a new normalcy and make it work for you.

It is because of her guidance and strength my whole life that I know I'm okay and will continue to be okay. We have great support to lean on when needed. My momma will not be suffering this lousy trial she was dealt at the end of her life. And as terrible as it will be to no longer have her alive on this earth, she will remain in my heart and mind as I continue my own path and my own journey.

She is just handing me her torch.

CHAPTER 86:
Through My Children's Eyes

October 24, 2022

I have two children who have journeyed through all of this.

When Mom was diagnosed back in 2020, she was already in her wheelchair. I remember the first time the kids came up to her house and saw her in it. I explained to them that Mamaw has a sickness called ALS that makes her body stop moving. My daughter had asked if she was going to get better. She was 8 at the time. My son, who was 4 at the time, believed Mamaw had COVID. I did my best to explain that Mamaw wouldn't get better, that she would in fact become more "sick" as time passed, and eventually she would go to Heaven—sooner than we all thought.

That's a lot for kids to digest. Heck, it's a lot for adults to digest.

Throughout that time, Mamaw didn't appear "sick," just "broken." Numerous times, my son would ask when she'd walk again, not fully understanding that she never would. Neither of them minded though, because Mamaw would sit them on her lap and give them rides up and down her street and around her house in her wheelchair.

When we made the decision to have Mom come live with us, I had more talks with the kids. I explained that Mamaw was getting worse with her ALS and that she needed us to take care of her. At this time, I did explain to them that Mamaw would live with us until she went to Heaven.

Then began a year and a half of ups and downs when it came to the kids and adjusting to Mom being here. My time with them was limited as I had to focus on taking care of Mom. I still did my best in being present with them, ensuring they got to do their activities, and having one-on-one time with them. There were many nights that they were asleep by the time I got Mom in bed, both already in dreamland before I'd had the chance to give them a kiss goodnight. Those nights hurt me.

As time went on, my daughter stayed up later and then began our "us" time after I put Mom in bed. We would watch shows together or just sit and be close to one another. There were also occasions when I used that time for "me" time, if at all possible.

My son, however, missed out on that. He was the one having the most difficult time with all of the changes that happened during the summer of 2021. We had moved into a new house, our dog of 12 years died, Mamaw moved in with us, and then he started kindergarten. Many times, he would speak his mind, stating that, "You never do anything with me anymore," and even, "I wish Mamaw never lived here." Talk about Mom Guilt times infinity. We had behavior issues with him during this time, but that also began to work itself out.

Things began to shift earlier this year. My son would often sit in the living room with Mom. Even though she was watching her shows and he was on his iPad, he was around her. With her. Near her. Often, he would be the one helping to tend to her needs. My daughter joined in some as well, especially when I had COVID, feeding her Mamaw for me.

Fast forward to last week.

I sat the kids down and explained what was happening. Reminding them of the conversation last year how Mamaw had come to live with us so that she'd be comfortable until it was her time to go to Heaven. I explained to them that the time had come, and she would soon be going.

My daughter was incredibly sad at first, but she told me she was crying more for me, because the thought of *me* dying was terrible so she knew me losing my own mom was going to make me so sad. My daughter has a heart of pure empathy.

My son hung his head down and I told him, "You know what, bub? When Mamaw goes to Heaven, she won't be in a wheelchair anymore. Isn't that great?"

My son stared at me and firmly said, "No, because she will be dead."

Yesterday, our incredible hospice nurse did a craft with the kids. She took mom's fingerprint and then theirs, putting them together like a heart, and had the kids decorate it and frame it. Before she started, she was talking with them, ensuring they understood what was happening to their Mamaw. Our nurse always has a smile on her face, she's just so phenomenally compassionate. My son, however, looked up at her with questioning eyes and asked, "Why are you smiling?" Because to my son, death is sad and not a happy time. He is very black-and-white in his thought processes.

When the nurse was leaving, she asked the kids if there was anything she could do for them or if they needed anything. My daughter smiled and asked jokingly if she'd take them to Disney World.

My son, who didn't smile, asked her, "Can you take my Mamaw to the hospital so that she can get better?" The nurse said she was sorry she couldn't do that, and my son's reply was, "Then there's nothing you can do for me." He is wise beyond his young years.

My son is having a harder time with this transition. They had both come to her side the last time she was conscious and told her they loved her, to which she was able to respond that she loved them too. That memory will forever be etched into my brain. My children were so brave. They understood they were saying their goodbyes and they didn't cry. They both smiled down at her, both held her hand and bent down to kiss her cheek. It took everything for me to hold in my own tears.

"I love you, sugars." Those were her last words to her grandchildren.

Without any prompting, my son drew her a picture. When he showed me, I almost lost it. It's a picture he drew of a single flower. He's come up with the phrase, *I love you in our hearts*, and stated he already missed her. He slept with his fingerprint craft last night.

This morning was rough getting them to school. My daughter, light hearted as she is, stopped in front of mom's closed bedroom door and told her she loved her. My son clung to me and cried. I hated taking him to school, but I wanted them to have some normalcy for now, if possible. I did contact the school for my son

207

and said if he was having any difficulties, I would come get him. I want to ensure my children's first real experience with death is one of understanding, sadness, celebration, and joy.

CHAPTER 87:
She Won

October 25, 2022

My Momma won her battle against ALS on October 25th, 2022.

Our journey together ended in the wee hours of the morning as I held her hand and told her I loved her over and over again.

She took her last breath and then joined my awaiting father.

Both of my parents have left this Earth.
Both at the age of 73.
Both in the month of October.

She left this world with elegance and grace, and I would have expected nothing less from the fierce little woman I called "Momma."

Though her journey has ended, mine will continue as I overcome my grief and learn to navigate life without my best friend beside me.

How is that even possible?

CHAPTER 88:
A Reflection of My "Why"

The act of writing about our journey together served many purposes. At first, it was a way for me to recollect how things transpired with her diagnosis and progression. ALS isn't as rare a diagnosis as you would think; however, it is not discussed as often as other diseases or ailments.

As we continued on, it became a way for me to express how I was feeling without the fear of being judged. I needed a way to release my stress without venting it toward the people in my life. My mother was always that one person I would call to vent about happenings in my life. When the things that needed venting were about her, well then, I needed somewhere else to turn.

The writing became public when we decided to share some tips and tricks for others dealing with ALS. It also allowed me to reach out to other caregivers of all ailments, to let them know that they're not alone. It became about support and connections.

I mention this because the details of what comes next—while vivid and personal in nature –are also meant to be educational. It's a reflection of the dying process, the grieving process, the journey of healing, and the rediscovery of self.

CHAPTER 89:
The Final Days

The last few days of her life were both educational and overwhelming—especially in a clinical sense. I witnessed things that I never knew were part of the dying process. I had worked in nursing homes for 18 years, but I had never stayed and watched each stage of the active dying process as it occurred.

At times it was so unnerving, even as hospice would try to explain it. Even being prepared, it will take you by surprise. The scents you smell was something I never knew about. There can be a "death smell" of a body as internal systems start to shut down. We had given Mom a complete bath just a day before she became bedbound. I continued to keep her clean, and yet there was this odor as I came into her room that would get worse as I leaned over her. When a catheter bag is emptied as a patient is dying, a very strong smell that is similar to rotting fruit comes from the urine. It's extremely potent. It helped to have a scented candle lit in the room. I'd like to think it made it more pleasant for visitors and for Momma too.

I'd heard the sounds known as the "death rattle" in the nursing homes. It was like a gurgling noise when the patient breathed in and out. What I didn't expect, nor had I ever heard before I witnessed it with my mom, was the moaning and grunting noise that is *very* loud and quite scary to hear. That is also noted to be the "death rattle," and once you hear it, you can never really *un*hear it.

The "3:30 syndrome" or developing a "Kennedy" is another part of the dying process I wasn't aware of, but thankfully the hospice nurse prepared me for it. When the body is shutting down, the blood goes where it's needed—to the heart, leaving all other organs to fend for themselves and shut down. This includes the body's biggest organ, the skin. Many times, a person will develop a bruise-like sore on their bottom that has a butterfly shape, within hours. That happened to mom. One morning her skin was perfect, and by that afternoon she had developed a Kennedy. Thankfully, people at this point are sedated enough with morphine that they don't necessarily feel the pain of this. Many I have talked with say this happens usually 24-48 hours before death. With Momma it was just a little over 24 hours after we found it that she took her last breath.

While all of this was unnerving, it was never horrifying or too much to take. It was explained very well thanks to our hospice nurses. Even with a clinical background in elder care, I wasn't aware of much of this, so it was very comforting to have it all explained that this was a natural process taking place. It's also why I include this for you. The more you are aware and can be prepared, the easier your journey can be.

CHAPTER 90

The Stillness After

Mom stayed in bed on a Wednesday due to fatigue. Her body was slowly shutting down, but she was able to talk, to visit, and to eat a few spoonfuls of broccoli cheddar soup. She was taking sips of water. Thursday was much of the same, and as Friday came, she was too tired to even get out of bed to use the bedside toilet, so a catheter was placed. On Saturday her fatigue was worse, and she spent more of the day sleeping than awake. Saturday was the last time she took any sips of water. On Sunday her CO_2 was climbing, yet she remained in little to no pain or distress. I began giving her the liquid morphine and Ativan to stay on top of it, and she again slept most of the day.

Monday morning was the last time Momma was conscious. In those few hours, before I'd give her the morphine at its due time, I rubbed her with lotion and moistened her lips. She smiled knowing I was there. Her voice was a slight whisper. She was able to tell me that she would always be with me. We had small, broken conversations that I knew would carry me through.

One of those little conversations revolved around my brother who was in jail. Throughout his years of troubles with addiction and the law, our mother was always there for him. Even when her other children told her to stop because we felt she was enabling him, she'd always tell us that he was her son. I never fully understood that until I had children of my own. Even in the final days of her life, Mom spoke out in her worry for him. She had said his name to me, and I knew exactly what she was telling me. I told her I'd take care of him, that I'd be there for him and not to worry. She smiled. I've kept that promise to her.

Momma's very last words to me before she fell into what would become her eternal sleep were, "I love you so much." It's the perfect last statement for anyone to hear. Although a few moments before

215

that I'd heard her whisper to no one particular "biscuits and gravy," which also would have been appropriate last words to me as well. Who doesn't love biscuits and gravy?

The rest of Monday, she never woke up as her body continued to fight. Fevers began as well as some wincing when the brain blocked and refused to accept the morphine. That's something else that is common to happen during the last days of life. Our brain processes pain medication, and for some reason it will start to block it. To correct this, a person has to be given increased doses closer together until the medicine can "break through" the block. This meant we had to give the pain meds to Mom about every 20 minutes until her body finally accepted the relief. This moment sticks out to me because giving someone that much pain medication can be very unnerving. I remember pausing during this phone discussion with the hospice nurse when she was giving me the directions on what to do. I will never, for the rest of my life, forget what she finally said to me that gave me the peace that I needed to continue.

"By doing this, you are *not* killing your mother. ALS is killing her. *You* are just making sure she is comfortable and not hurting. *You* are giving her relief."

Although now in a coma, her body continued to fight and would just not give up. Me and my siblings, along with her life partner, continued to kiss her forehead and tell her it was okay to go.

However, she wasn't listening to us. Go figure. Even with death, she was being stubborn.

Late Monday night, I was in the den with my daughter, looking through photos as we prepared the visitation "funeral boards" with memories of Mom. My daughter had asked me why Mamaw hadn't gone to Heaven yet, and I explained to her that we didn't know. We'd all given her permission to, but she just hadn't yet. My daughter asked me if she could try. I was stunned and taken aback. The kids had said their "I love yous" one night before bed when Mom was conscious and alert. I hadn't brought them into her room since.

My daughter wanted to go in now though, so I took her inside Mom's room. She stood next to the bed and smiled down at her sleeping grandma. My daughter talked to her. She told her that it was okay to go to Heaven now, because she'd be with Papaw and Bailey (Mom's dog that passed), her own parents, Jesus, and God. She kissed her grandma's forehead and smiled down at her once more. She then fearlessly and gracefully walked out of Mom's room. The swell of admiration and love I felt as I watched my young daughter do this is something I could never put into words and that I will always remember.

We went back to the den to finish photos on the boards, and about twenty minutes later, Momma started the death rattle. I ushered my daughter to bed so that she wouldn't hear it. Another thirty minutes, and Momma's vitals started to fall.

I slept on my mother's bedroom floor that night, drifting in and out of sleep as we listened to Vince Gill's, "*Go Rest High on that Mountain,*" play on an endless loop. About 4 a.m., I awoke to stand and check on her. I noticed Momma's breathing was short. I held her hand, looking down at her. I told her I loved her. She then took two final breaths.

Momma was released.

I didn't cry at that moment. She looked so beautiful and elegant. You often hear stories of people passing away and their muscles causing their eyes to open or their body releases. Not my momma though. She looked as if she were just sleeping. She looked comfortable and relaxed as she left us.

I sat with her for some time, humming along with the song that continued to play as memories flashed through my mind. I closed my eyes and saw her standing over the oven cooking. I saw that smile of hers reach her eyes and her head tilt back laughing. I saw her holding each of my children as babies the day they were born. I envisioned her arms wrapped around me as a child, breathing in the "Momma smell" of her favorite perfume.

Opening my eyes, I kissed her on her forehead and left her room to start making the calls and getting started on what needed to be done. At this point I still hadn't cried. The hospice nurse and one of Momma's caregivers came over to prepare her to be taken away. The funeral home came in the dark of early morning. I stood in the den as they wheeled her out of her room and toward the door. A lump in my throat started to form, but I swallowed it away, leaning over to kiss her and watch as her body was taken away.

People came and went. Calls and texts were made and answered. In the later morning, my siblings went with me to the funeral home to make preparations. When I came home, the gates of emotions finally bolted open, and I wept.

I wept.
I wept.
I wept.

I wept harder than I ever had in my entire life. Ugly sobs and moans, calling out for my Momma, as the pain seemed to squeeze my heart until it was going to explode. The waves of grief were monumental in size and power. I'd never experienced anything like it.

I was not only grieving the loss of my mother, but I feel as though the waves also held insurmountable volumes of relief and reality as they pummeled my body. The relief that the journey was done—my duties had been relieved. The reality that my momma was gone—I'd never talk to her again, never see her again. The reality that I was an orphan now—even at almost 40 years old, that's a tough pill to swallow.

Mom had died on a Tuesday. That entire day was hard. Hard doesn't even cover it, but it was also very busy and there wasn't a lot of down time. Except at night. For the first time in 15 months, I went to bed without a baby monitor next to me. I felt like a part of me was missing, because it was.

Wednesday, all the family started to arrive, and our house was full. There was a lot to be done, and we were kept busy. Having everyone around helped to keep the agony at bay. I would comfort others as they broke. I would laugh and smile as memories were shared. I'd hold it together, until the night came.

Thursday was her funeral viewing. I stood beside her casket with my husband and siblings by my side for four hours as family and friends came to pay their final respects to Mom. I held it together well except when a friend that I share with my brother, who was in jail, came through the line. Hugging her was just a reminder that he wasn't there. I broke slightly and told her I needed him, which in turn got her to break down as well.

Friday, we laid her to rest alongside my father. The service was beautiful. The Nursing Honor Guard came from the hospital and did a ceremony. It was something my mother would have loved. It was during that moment that I almost broke. Almost. I held it together though. I stayed strong and was as resilient as I knew my mother would have wanted me to be.

Saturday, everyone went home. My extended family had to return to their own lives. It was then that I had waves of grief strike me multiple times. I no longer had others to keep me occupied. It had been a whirlwind of a week with so many people here, and now the quiet came. The unavoidable quiet that follows heightened events.

The "new normal" was beginning, and reality crept back in. I slept most of that Saturday afternoon. That evening I went out to eat with my husband and kids, something we hadn't casually done since 2019, before COVID struck and Momma moved in. We took the kids to a Halloween Trunk or Treat and then to their only remaining grandparent's house to stay the night.

Grief came when I knew Momma would have loved to see them dressed up. Grief came when we dropped them off at my husband's mothers house, knowing I was returning to an empty house. It's been odd for me to be cautious about going into public. Not because I'll break down when I see people I know, but because the grief strikes me after seeing them.

I know I have to get on with my life and continue to move. Momma's words, "suck it up and deal," are true to this cause as well. I'm allowing myself to feel the grief, but I refuse to live in it.

My momma's pain is no more. Only mine is just beginning. I am surrounded with memories and love, as well as with my family by my side, to guide me through.

Our journey together is done, but a new journey now begins. A new chapter in life as I continue to carry the torch she so brightly lit and has now passed on to me.

CHAPTER 91:
Crashing Waves of Grief

November 2, 2022

I returned to work today.

Transitioning into this new chapter that no longer physically includes my mother is not an easy chapter to begin. It's odd for me to experience depression, grief, and anxiety because I've never dealt with these feelings all at once like I am doing now.

When my father passed away 10 years ago, I remember one breakdown I had where I laid in bed and sobbed for a good half an hour as my husband held me. I didn't cry at his showing, but I did during the funeral (military funerals are rough). I don't remember the huge crashing of waves that carried tons of emotions with them, not like these.

I suppose it is because I had my mother to focus on during and after that time. I felt the responsibility to guard her against her own grief and depression and fully invest myself in her happiness after we lost him. I would cry at every holiday for a couple years after he died. Always a short cry in the mornings before I began Thanksgiving cooking or before waking the kids to see what Santa had brought.

Perhaps I figured this time would be much like that. Only, it isn't.

I had thought to myself throughout the time Mom lived with us that her passing would be sad, of course. But the relief that not only her journey had ended, but ours as well, would uplift the grief in some form of joy for her and for all of us.

It hasn't.

Instead, when her pain ended, mine enhanced to the point of explosion. Although I remained strong (and perhaps in shock) during her visitation and her funeral, I sobbed guttural agony before those days and have quite frequently since.

I got up around 1:00 a.m. to use the restroom last night, and when I lay back down, I had trouble falling asleep. Her face was in the forefront of my mind. Out of nowhere, a wave of grief struck, and I spent the next 20 minutes sobbing into my pillow before sleep welcomed me back to peace.

Today I went back to work (physically, as I'd been working from home), and I prepared myself for the looks of sympathy, the hugs and words of comfort. I did receive those, but there weren't waves or even ripples of grief. Instead, I busied myself.

It was when I l*eft* work. A twisted ball of nerves settled in the pit of my stomach. My chest began to feel tight and heavy. As I drove to pick up my son from after-school care, it worsened. By the time the two of us pulled into our driveway, I was near a full-blown panic attack.

It didn't amount to that, thankfully. I knew if I began to break down with just my son and I at home that I would possibly scare him. It was a blessing that my husband got off work early today and was home soon after us.

My husband hugged me, and I melted into another wave that I'd been holding in since I left work. I finally broke down and took something so I could function. There is no shame in that.

It was yet another first—the first time I came home from the most "normal" day since she aspirated. I came home to a house where she was no longer waiting for me. I'm aware enough to realize that, soon enough, the "firsts" will decrease. I'm not saying the pain of her absence will get any easier. I just know that it will hurt "differently."

One day the pain won't constantly take my breath away or make me feel sick to my stomach. One day the thought that my Momma is gone from this Earth won't seem like such an absurdity. The reality will take hold, and I will continue on just as I had with my father.

I have missed my father since he left us 10 years ago.
I will forever miss him.

I will forever miss my momma.

Even knowing my family and I did everything possible to ensure she was cared for and loved here at home. Even though I know she was thankful and proud of me. Even though I am proud of myself. Even with all of that…

…the waves continue to crash into me.

CHAPTER 92:
A Final Letter to You

November 19, 2022

Dear Momma,

It's been almost a month since you took your last breath. We have had so many memories and so many moments between us in my 40 years as your daughter. The moments leading up to you physically leaving me will forever be cherished and will forever swallow me in grief, all at the same time.

This past week, I went to Florida like I planned for a work conference. It was something I had begun planning and scheduling this spring, knowing I would need caregivers 24/7 for those five days I would be gone in November. I tried not to stress about it, and when I *did* stress, I tried to make sure *you* could never tell. I'm sure you did, though. You knew me better than I knew myself. Part of me believes you left when you did, *on purpose*.

My heart broke picking up my phone to call or text you to tell you about the great workshops I attended, to tell you the sites I got to see, and to listen to your advice because my son became really sick while I was far from home.

My heart broke because you physically were not there. I savored the beautiful Florida sunrise and sunset, closing my eyes and feeling your presence surround me in those moments. I smiled, and then I sobbed.

I don't want to *feel* your presence, Mom.

I don't want to talk to you in my head or reach for your strength in my heart. I want to *feel you*. I want to smell my "Momma Smell." I want to see that smile of yours touch your eyes as I make you laugh.

I selfishly want *you*.

Here.
With Me.

I don't have you physically here anymore. You are now free of that terrible ALS monster you fought and finally broke away from.

You are walking.
You are dancing.
You are laughing.
You are *whole*.
Your pain ended, and mine truly began.

Oh, I try to stay strong. I have done well for the most part lately. However, coming home brings back the rough reality that it's empty of you. Yet, it's so full of you all at the same time.

I'm preparing for Thanksgiving here at the house. We will be taking down the fall decor next weekend and getting out the Christmas decorations.

Your Christmas decorations.

I'll be putting out all your deer and Santa's that you loved so much. Your white Christmas tree you were so proud of and sat looking at all last year—that's going right where you liked having it.

Today turned into an emotional day for me, and I know so many more are to follow. I'm trying my best to keep going, to continue forward. Some days I am great, and other days I am not. I have yet to cook a meal for my family since you've been gone. I've just been in a slump and feel like I'm a 'bump on a log'. I catch myself sitting and staring into space as I'm lost in memories of you.

Funny how when you were here with me, cooking was what soothed me and gave me *my* time. I'd spend time in the kitchen just to have moments of clarity and be away from everyone needing me. Now that I have all that time, cooking has been the last thing I have wanted to do. I've got to work toward changing that. I've got to work toward moving on and focus on my life again with my family.

I am going to.
I have to be better – you taught me to be better.
I miss you, Momma.

Words cannot even describe the emptiness I feel without you here with me. I am surrounded by so much support, loving family, and cherished friends. My husband is such a blessing and is taking such good care of me. You'd be so proud of that.

Yet, I feel so alone, Momma.

How is it you're gone?
How?
How in this world can anything exist without you in it?

You were my *best* friend, Momma. You still are and you always will be.

There is no more strife—just a lifetime of gratitude.

I love you.
I love you more.
Impossible.

Cassie